If you do external exercises,
you *must* do internal exercises.
If you do internal exercises,
you may forget to practice external exercises!

THE
BOOK
OF
INTERNAL
EXERCISES

Dr. Stephen T. Chang
with
Richard C. Miller

Photography by Peter M. Cornwell

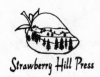

Strawberry Hill Press

Strawberry Hill Press
2594–15th Avenue
San Francisco, California 94127

Manufactured in the United States of America

Edited by Scott Lowe

Book design by Carlton Clark Herrick

Library of Congress Cataloging in Publication Data

Chang, Stephen Thomas, 1935-
    The book of internal exercises.

    1. Exercise.   2. Hygiene, Taoist,   3. Vitality.
I. Miller, Rick, 1948-   joint author.   II. Title
III. Title: Internal exercises.
RA781.C47   613.7   78-18320
ISBN 0-89407-017-7

*TO THE SPIRIT
THAT LIES WITHIN THE HEART
OF EACH OF US*

Acknowledgments

The authors wish to acknowledge and thank the following:

Denise Lowe, for her patience, understanding, kindness, and poses.

Ku, Fu-sheng, for his additional art work — and gentle counsel.

The College of San Mateo, Golden West College, and Marin School of Yoga for their assistance during the lecture presentations from which this book developed.

Maryann and Paul Pearson for their kind help and support.

And Cat and Chuck for their loving company — "they sat with me when I needed them!"

About the Authors

Stephen Thomas Chang's grandmother was a master-physician, while her father was both personal physician to Empress Chih Shee and the first Chinese ambassador to the United Kingdom. Dr. Chang has been trained in both Chinese and Western medicine, and in addition to his medical degrees he holds degrees in law, philosophy, and theology. A Taoist, he lectures world-wide on various aspects of Taoism, and he is the author of *The Complete Book of Acupuncture* (Celestial Arts, 1976).

Richard Cushing Miller, who has his M.A. in group dynamics and human relations from San Francisco State University, is Director of the Marin School of Yoga. He is an acknowledged master of Hatha Yoga, doing his doctoral work at the California Institute of Asian Studies in the psychology of Yoga, and is particularly interested in the relationship of Taoism to the principles of Yoga.

Contents

List of Photographs, Figures and Illustrations

Photographs:

There is a thing inherent and natural
Which existed before heaven and earth
Motionless and fathomless,
It stands alone and never changes;
It pervades everywhere and never becomes exhausted.
It may be regarded as the Mother of the Universe.
I do not know its name.
If I am forced to give it a name,
I call it Tao, and I name it as supreme.
Supreme means going on,
Going on means going far,
Going far means returning.
Therefore Tao is supreme; heaven is supreme;
     earth is supreme; and man is also supreme.
     There are in the universe four things supreme,
     and man is one of them.
Man follows the laws of earth;
Earth follows the laws of heaven;
Heaven follows the laws of Tao;
Tao follows the laws of its intrinsic nature.

                    Tao Te Ching, XXV

Introduction

The Book of Internal Exercises is not about Taoism, but it is impossible to consider the exercises apart from their Taoist origination. Taoism is the eldest of the world's religions. It is said in legend that Lao-tzu, the best-known and perhaps the greatest of Taoist sages, "transformed" himself, or incarnated again as Sakyamuni Buddha. The Tao Te Ching itself is primarily a political treatise and a theoretical representation of Taoism expressed from the point of view of an elightened being. The formulation of the practical and functional aspects was left to other Taoist sages. And so it was that the ancient Chinese masters devised, in addition to the basic spiritual doctrines and philosophy of Taoism, innumerable techniques designed to ultimately transform and immortalize the physical body. Moreover, these techniques have been known and practiced for the past 6,000 years in the Orient, but they have been kept secret from the West until the present time.

The Internal Exercises themselves are one part of a four-fold system of Taoist thought and practice. The four pillars of Taoism are the I Ching, Sexology, Diet and the Internal Exercises. The focus of this book is necessarily then upon the Internal Exercises, but they must be seen in their larger context before they may be properly understood. And so before we begin examining the exercises in detail, we will attempt to summarize the four pillars that uphold the living structure which is Taoism.

THE I CHING

The I Ching is a system of wisdom which enables us to direct our everyday actions; it is comprised of astrology, philosophy, and various techniques of forecasting. The study of the I Ching is divided into three parts:

The first is a study of symbols or signs representing the phenomena of endless changes occurring throughout the universe. The phenomena of universal change are governed by exact laws defined by the various branches of mathematics — algebra, geometry, physics and genetics.

The second section is the study of social philosophy and transactional psychology, as represented by the 64 hexagrams. Each hexagram is composed of six lines, of which each line represents a developing stage in individual or group transactions.

The third part of study is the actual practice of forecasting events. Everything that has happened is going to happen again, and everything that is going to occur has occurred already. ("Going on means going far,/ Going far means returning. . . .") It is therefore possible for us to predict the future if we understand the I Ching.

1

TAOIST SEXOLOGY

Taoism was the first religion to take human sexuality fully into account, to present it in such a way that people could use their sexual energy to transform themselves. (The Hindus too were sophisticated in this regard, as is evidenced by the *Kama Sutra*, a treatise written in approximately the 7th Century A.D., which set forth rules for sexual behavior and marriage in accordance with Hindu law.) Taoist sexology directs people so they can enjoy sexual play without depleting themselves, explains how to strengthen the sexual organs and how to use sexual energy to cure specific ailments, elucidates various positions of therapeutic intercourse, natural birth control, and eugenics — including ways to select the sex of your child.

DIET

The system of diet is divided into three categories. The first category is the food diet, which explains in detail which foods are best to eat, the therapeutic properties of various foods, and how to combine foods into tasteful and attractive dishes. The food diet also includes a detailed analysis of various ingredients contained in foods, the acid and alkaline content of foods, along with the correct way to balance vitamins, minerals and proteins. What we eat is of utmost importance; regardless of how well we have learned any other discipline, if we eat poison, we will surely die. The system of diet is the product of 6,000 years of meticulous observation. Interestingly enough, the basic principles, insofar as using natural and unprocessed foods, have remained virtually the same throughout all this time.

The second category of the diet is the herbal diet, which takes us one step beyond the food diet. A proverb of Chinese medicine is that "Food is medicine and medicine should be food." Even though one may live in accordance with the principles of the food diet, it is still possible for harmful bacteria to thrive within the body — for just as we derive a certain amount of our energy from food, harmful bacteria are also able to multiply by the energy they derive from that same food. To remedy this apparent dilemma, the ancient Taoists formulated what is generally known as Chinese herbology.

Herbs are easily and totally assimilated by the body. Consequently, their therapeutic values are unsurpassed. (It is interesting to note in this context, that in Revelations 22:2 it is written, "The leaves of the tree were for the healing of the nation.") Along with being able to purify the body and act as antibiotics against germs, herbs can also greatly increase our energy level and life span. The herbal category of diet is therefore indispensible in reaching our goal of superb physical health and even physical immortality.

The third category is the energy diet. It is similar in nature to energy breathing, which is described in a later chapter of this book. When one reaches the level of energy breathing, food and herbs are no longer necessary because the body is nourished directly by cosmic energy. There have been many instances of this achievement, but no doubt the best-known example of energy breathing is the story of Jesus' forty-day sojourn in the wilderness. He abstained from food and water during that time, being nourished directly by Spirit, the universal force or energy. Because cosmic energy is the same whether one is on Earth, Mars or in the outer reaches of the galaxy, Taoist adepts strive to transform and attune their bodies to a degree whereby they can travel to any part of the universe, and be nourished by that all-pervading energy.

INTERNAL EXERCISES

The Internal Exercises are the very opposite of external exercises. While external exercises such as swimming, boxing, wrestling, weight lifting, tennis, kung-fu and karate may produce an attractive outer figure, they often do so by depleting the energy of the internal organs, thereby causing not only any number of illnesses, but also premature aging. Internal exercises, on the other hand, are designed to energize the entire body, balance the energy level, and promote a more effective functioning of the internal organs.

The Internal Exercises are an expression of the art of self-healing. If one goes against the laws of nature, illness will result. If one never has a mild illness, then a serious disease will never develop; if one never has a serious disease, one will not die, for death is believed to be the end result of the accumulation of many illnesses throughout one's lifetime. To be totally free of disease, however, does not guarantee a state of physical immortality, for the body must be able to accomodate the influx of additional energy which in the end will transform it into a vehicle unconditioned by time and space. It is because the Internal Exercises meet these dual requirements that they form the foundation of Taoism. The Internal Exercises are divided into three categories.

The first category contains exercises designed to teach correct posture and the proper way to sit, recline, walk and work. Thousands of years ago, Chinese sages selected three animals that were noted for longevity; they minutely observed the behavior that seemed to contribute to their longevity. The three basic Internal Exercises are:

(a) The Deer Exercise, which is designed to generate and balance the secretions of the endocrine glands.

(b) The Crane Exercise, which is designed to strengthen the organs within the trunk of the body. Even though these organs are controlled by the autonomic nervous system, the Crane Exercise enables one to balance the energy and promote thereby a smoother functioning among these organs.

(c) The Turtle Exercise, which is designed to aid one in strengthening, relaxing, and eventually controlling the entire nervous system.

In addition to the preceding, there are other exercises designed to strengthen the limbs, muscles and bones. It usually takes three months to become proficient in these exercises. The important point to make here,

3

however, is that self-healing, which is the natural result of doing these exercises on a regular basis, is guaranteed.

The second category of the Internal Exercises is called Meridian Meditation, Trip-Around-The-World Meditation, or simply, Taoist Contemplation. The pathways for circulation of energy throughout the body are called meridians. Thus, Meridian Meditation is a technique to stimulate the flow of energy along these pathways and to simultaneously balance the energy within the body. In affirming that man is the microcosm and that the universe is the macrocosm, we must go on to say that it is necessary to unify the two. Through meditation, first the body, mind and intellect become totally and consciously integrated. The next phase is one in which the individual becomes inseparably and totally enlivened by cosmic or universal energy. Both acupuncture and acupressure are generally utilized for the benefit of others. Following the initial training, Meridian Meditation takes anywhere from six months to ten years of practice.

The third category of the Internal Exercises is Cosmic Breathing or Energy Breathing. These are exercises whereby energy is absorbed through the acupuncture points which lie atop the meridians that traverse the body. Energy is being constantly depleted through daily living, and so it is necessary to replenish our energy supply in order to ward off weakness, disease and death. Energy Breathing is therefore a vital step in self-healing and in forming an indivisible link with the energy permeating the universe. As in Meridian Meditation, Energy Breathing requires anywhere from six months to ten years of practice to perfect.

The four-fold system of which Taoism is comprised covers every aspect of our everyday existence. It is designed to completely nourish our basic physical needs in such a manner that we can progress slowly but steadily with an ever-growing confidence in knowing that we shall one day reach our cherished goal. The heartwarming benefits so immediately reaped from a sincere and selfless application of any of the exercises are enough to instill within us a kind of fervor, which of itself will move us forward along the path.

So-called spiritual development should not have to be chased after — it should be the natural result of our everyday actions. It is not necessary to stress spiritual life or to be concerned with the state of our souls, for the divine is pure and everywhere existent; it has always been so and shall always be. Rather, we should be concerned with our physical bodies and how we can use the time we do have to get beyond the degenerating aspect of time, joyfully striving every minute of the day to reach that level where we too can live in the Tao.

1 The Theory of Energy

The root of the way of life, of birth and change is Qi (energy); the myriad things of heaven and earth all obey this law. Thus Qi in the periphery envelops heaven and earth. Qi in the interior activates them. The source where-from the sun, moon, and stars derive their light, the thunder, rain, wind and cloud their being, the four seasons and the myriad things their birth, growth, gathering and storing: all this is brought about by Qi. Man's possession of life is completely dependent upon this Qi.

Nei Ching

The ancient Chinese texts, expounding on the basic theories that energy supported all life and matter in the cosmos, were written to convey basic scientific principles in a style that attracted the attention of even those who were not inclined toward a serious study of science. This is not to imply that the barriers between the artistic, scientific and practical ways of life were as distinct and offered such a marked degree of specialization as are those characterizing modern civilization. The integrated man, as he existed in ancient China, was one who constantly strove to maintain a balance between the various modes of life — the artistic, the scientific and the practical. It was no great effort for the scientist to record his observations in a style which today would be called "poetic" in form — it came to him naturally. That scientific principles could be conveyed in such imaginative form attests to the unification of art and science which typifies the Golden Age of Chinese civilization.

It may well be that because the basic principles of Chinese medical science are poetically stated, many modern scientists choose to reject them, avowing them to be "unscientific," "purely philosophical," "mystical," and "primitive." But the rejection of traditional principles on these grounds, far from indicating a greater degree of objective awareness on the part of the modern day men of science, suggests instead a growing gap between science and a true "art of living." The principles of Chinese medical science and the Internal Exercise system as they have come down through the ages are just as applicable today as they were in the past, but they must be interpreted through a proper understanding of the poetic form that has enshrined and carried them through the ages.

THE NATURE OF ENERGY

Energy is a dynamic force, in constant flux, which circulates throughout the body. Many people plausibly substitute the word *life* for the word *energy* since the essential difference between the two words is so subtle that it eludes all but the semanticist. Each term is vital to developing an accurate understanding of the energy theory as it applies to the body.

For all practical purposes, it can be stated that life is an *indication* of energy within the body. All that comes to mind on hearing the word *life* — breathing, talking, sleeping, eating, even the ability to read, think, and hear — all these can be achieved only because of the energy within the body. This invariably applies to those functions or activities that are not conspicuously perceptible; for example, the metabolic processes within each single cell could not be accomplished without energy to sustain those functions. Energy is the basis for the apparent solid structures of the body and all that pertains to its anatomy as well. For what is a solid structure such as a bone, except a mass of living cells? All forms and activities of life, both anatomical and physiological, are supported by, and simultaneously deplete, the energy within the body.

Although most people assume that inert matter is completely solid or dense, it is energy which binds the protrons, electrons and neutrons within each individual atom. Inanimate matter, then, is simply energy at a different rate of vibration than that of other forms of life. *Energy therefore is the absolute basis for all forms of life and matter in the universe.*

Developing a comprehension of energy and all that pertains to a scientific mode of its expression — in this case, within and as the human body — enables an adept practitioner of acupuncture to initiate the so-called miracles traditionally ascribed to this ancient science. Being thoroughly acquainted with the precise manner in which energy exists within the body, an experienced practitioner can beneficently manipulate this most subtle, all-pervading force. Since energy supports all vital functions associated with the body, the ability to adjust that energy enables one to regulate those functions which that energy supports; in an identical manner, dysfunctions or diseases of the body can be eliminated by readjusting the energy imbalance that is the unseen cause of the apparent dysfunction. A person placidly undergoing major surgery while remaining fully conscious under the influence of acupunctural anaesthesia is a perfect example of what an understanding of energy, and how it enlivens the body, enables a practitioner to do.

Food and air are considered to be the primary sources of energy depleted through daily living rather than as fuel to be metabolized by the body. Energy, though, is not obtained from the gross molecular aspects of food and air, but rather from what can be called its "vibrational" essence, or, its electromagnetism. For instance: The nutrients within any particular food can be accurately reproduced in a biochemist's laboratory, but life cannot be sustained over a prolonged period of time by ingesting those synthetic nutrients alone; it is possible to obtain every single vitamin, mineral, and chemical that comprises an egg, and yet it is impossible to

6

transform them into anything that vaguely resembles a genuine egg. Neither is a person able to exist over a prolonged period of time on pure oxygen which has been obtained by laboratory methods, or in a room in which the air has been filtered by an electrical air-conditioner. In all of these instances something is lacking, and that "something" is the particular object's *life essence,* its electromagnetism — that invisible energy which enlivens gross molecular aspects of any object.

Electromagnetism is a force with which most of us are not yet familiar. It was Western scientists who ingeniously verified the existence of electromagnetism, providing thereby a means for the logical explanation for many of the previously unexplained phenomena resulting from acupuncture therapy, as well as the health enhancing benefits obtained through practice of the Internal Exercises. In short, electromagnetism is an intensity force that permeates the atomic structures of all objects, including the surrounding atmosphere. Because it is a natural force, it has a rapport with the energy within the body. When needles are inserted into the skin during an acupuncture treatment, they act as antennae that conduct the electromagnetic energy from the air into the body. Similarly, the Internal Exercises work to stimulate the body's natural abilities to replenish the energy depleted through daily living.

THE MERIDIANS

Energy circulates throughout the body along minute pathways called *meridians.* An understanding of the meridians and their vital function of providing every cell of the body with energy is mandatory if one is to master the techniques of the breathing and contemplation exercises in the system of Internal Energizing Exercises.

> *The means whereby man is created, the means whereby diseases occur, the means whereby man is cured, the means whereby diseases arise: the twelve meridians are the basis for all theory and treatment. The meridian is that which decides over life and death. Through it the hundred diseases may be treated.*
> Nei Ching

Regarding the meridians, Dr. Kim Bong Han of the University of Pyongang in North Korea, after conducting an extensive series of experiments, arrived at a conclusion for the actual existence of these pathways of energy. He reported that the meridians were actually composed of a type of histological tissue as yet unnoticed by scientists who, prior to Dr. Kim's experiments, had believed that the meridians were simply *imaginary* lines. He discovered the structure and function of the meridian system to be totally different from those of the lymphatic, circulatory, and nervous systems.

The meridians are symmetrical and bilateral channels with a diameter ranging between 20 and 50 millimicrons. They exist beneath the surface of the skin and have a thin membranous wall which is filled with a transparent, colorless fluid. Each of the main meridians develops intricate subsidiary branches, some of which supply adjacent areas with energy while others ultimately reach the surface of the skin. The places at which the branches reach the skin's surface are the points illustrated on an acupuncture chart. Often several branches from different main channels converge at a single point. By stimulating that point, the energy in several channels can be affected simultaneously. The meridians are encircled by blood vessels that are especially in abundance around the individual branches stemming from each of the main channels. The phenomenon of bleeding that some patients report after undergoing acupuncture is an indication that the practitioner has narrowly missed the point on the surface of the skin and pierced one or many of the vascular vessels surrounding the point.

After conducting many experiments, scientists discovered that the meridians are pathways for electricity. This led to the invention of a machine called the Point-Locator, an instrument which indicates the points where the branches of the meridians reach the skin's surface. At present the quality of the impulse that travels along the meridians is the subject of intensive research among Chinese scientists, while many Western investigators are currently trying to determine possible associations between the meridians and the autonomic nervous system.

The meridian system, a physiological structure, provides a means by which many of the energy principles that have been labeled as purely hypothetical — even to the point where their actual existence has been questioned — can be proved valid. Since the reality of the meridian system has been experimentally verified by researchers like Dr. Kim, we can now conclude that the main functional purpose for which that system exists is to provide an effective means of transmission for that all-pervading but invisible energy which animates all manifestations of life. Their delicate subtlety, when perceived in relationship to even the most microscopic aspects of the gross physical body, suggests that the meridians may well be the "missing link," or the threshold between pure energy and its first manifestations as microscopic matter.

"Meridian" is a word borrowed from geography, indicating a line joining a series of ordered points. There are twelve main meridians — one assigned to each of the five organs, the six bowels, and the pericardium — here referred to as the heart constrictor. (The idea of the six bowels is often perplexing to those unacquainted with Chinese medicine and philosophy. The five organs are the heart, spleen-pancreas, lungs, kidneys and liver. The six bowels are the large intestine, bladder, "triple heater" (an ancient term indicating the internal glandular system), gallbladder, small intestine and stomach. The heart constrictor or pericardium corresponds to the blood vessel system. (Please refer to my book *The Complete Book of Acupuncture* for a fuller explanation.)

Although the first scientific proof of the existence of the meridian system is believed to be the result of Dr. Kim's efforts, conclusive evidence for the existence of the meridians was actually found in 1937 by Sir Thomas Lewis of England. His report, published in the *British Medical Journal* of February, 1937, stated he had discovered an "unknown nervous system" that was unrelated to either the sensory or the sympathetic nervous systems. Rather than being composed of a network of nerves, he reported, the newly discovered system was composed of a network of incredibly minute lines. Although his report went relatively unnoticed by his colleagues, it was the first concrete verification in the West of the physiological system that Chinese medicine knew to exist thousands of years ago.

THE POINTS OF ENTRY AND EXIT

Each of the main meridians has both a point of entry and a point of exit. Energy enters the meridian at the point of entry, circulates along the meridian, flows through the point of exit and on through the point of entry of the succeeding meridian. The point of exit on a meridian is connected to the point of entry on the succeeding meridian by a secondary channel. The direction of the flow of energy along a meridian remains constant and never vacillates after flowing through the point of entry.

The meridians are the means by which the organs and bowels are linked together, and by which each organ and bowel is enlivened by energy as it circulates along the meridian circuit. A question that might naturally arise as a result of the illustrations depicting the sequence of the main meridians is: "According to the information given thus far — if an organ or bowel associated with one of the main meridians were to become diseased, wouldn't it be logical to conclude that the energy would then be blocked and unable to complete its cycle of circulation?" The answer to this is no, because in addition to the twelve main meridians, there are eight extraordinary meridians which provide for the circulation of energy when it becomes superfluous or excessive in one of the main meridians.

The eight extraordinary meridians can justifiably be called "life-savers" in that they provide for bodily energy to continue its cycle of circulation regardless of whether any one of the organs or bowels becomes diseased, thus blocking the meridian circuit. Traditional Chinese Medicine explains the purpose of the eight extraordinary meridians as being analogous to the drainage ditches and dikes that sometimes exist alongside a major river (which, of course, corresponds to the major meridians). If for any reason the river should become flooded and overflow its banks, the drainage ditches are designed to accommodate the superfluous water. Just so, the flow of energy along the eight extraordinary meridians is not constant, but is determined by the amount of excess energy in a main meridian.

INTERNAL EXERCISES

The efficacy of the Internal Exercises is based on the development of the proper flow of energy throughout the meridians in the body. Each exercise is designed to stimulate a particular meridian, or, as in the case of the Meridian Meditation, the entire meridian system. By learning the Internal Energizing Exercises, we are able to gain control over the very energy upon which all life depends. We can then use this energy to heal both ourselves and others, and to insure our continuing health and spiritual growth and even our potential immortality.

2 The Deer, The Crane and The Turtle

The Deer, the Crane and the Turtle form the foundation which supports the Taoist Art of Chi-Kung or Internal Energizing Exercises. These three, and the other exercises presented here, were arrived at by ancient Taoists through careful study of the natural principles of healing. When combined with the meditative and breathing techniques, they make up a wonderful self-healing system. When followed daily, they promote not only freedom from disease and pain, but a wonderful sense of well-being which springs from the heart of the individual. They represent a step which any conscientious person can easily take toward a transformation of the body from the material to the eternal. The Chinese recognized that not everyone would undergo such a transformation during their existing lifetime. However, they emphasized that one still needed to follow these exercises on a daily basis so that one could at the very least obtain perfect health and happiness during one's lifetime. They felt that each man and woman had the right to live a life free of physical pain, mental disharmony and spiritual selfishness. At a time when most people can only look forward to growing old with a sense of trepidation, this system of Internal Exercises represents an exciting turning point.

Stress — environmental, social and internal — breeds fear and disease. Presently, growing old conjures up images of high blood pressure, arteriosclerosis, embolisms, cancers and diseases of all imaginable types. Until recently, Westerners have been given few alternatives for dealing with these stresses. We have allowed our bodies and minds to weaken with only cursory hopes of slowing the aging process and deterring disease for a time. However the main emphasis of the Internal Exercises *is on strengthening our bodies and minds.* They aim to tone all the internal systems, including the emotional and the spiritual. By performing these simple exercises on a daily basis, we can look forward to growing old with a sense of ease and excitement, knowing we carry with us from year to year an inner sense of vitality and aliveness which comes only from living a life free from the anxiety of future illnesses and the weakness due to present diseases. Only when we have developed this sense of freedom and this inner vitality will we be able to create a fertile ground upon which our true spiritual nature can unfold. And only then can we attempt to reach out for the transformation of our material bodies into the eternal.

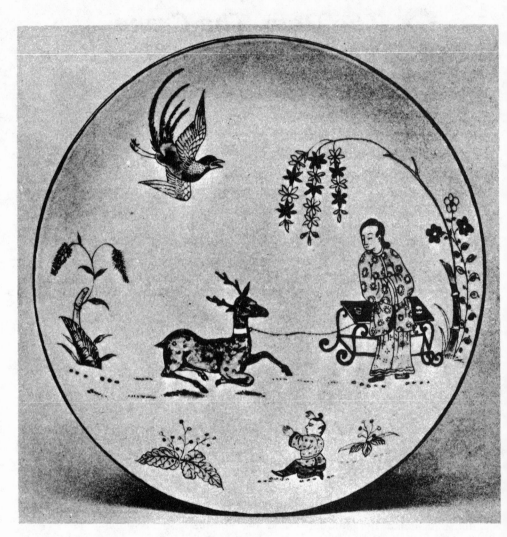

The Deer

A state of harmony brings with it a feeling that there is no good or bad, positive or negative, Yin or Yang, disease or fear. When a shoulder heals, one often has to be reminded that at one time it suffered great pain. When one reaches this point, it is easy to stop practicing all exercises. Thus one may inadvertently fall back into weakness and disease. One needs, then, an outer sense of discipline at first to continue to pursue this, as is necessary in any endeavor. We hope, however, that an inner sense of discipline will develop within the practitioner which will carry him or her forward on a continual movement of interest. This movement arises from the understanding, growth and feeling of wellness which comes from following these Internal Exercises.

The Internal Exercises are easily performed, require no strenuous activity, and do not require a great amount of time to perform. They are a gift to the Western world from the ancient Taoists, and when used wisely and with a feeling of appreciation, will be well worth the time and energy invested in practicing them. They have been developed around natural laws of healing, and therefore one need not be in a hurry to "master" them. Take your time in developing a feeling for each exercise and you will be rewarded with ample treasures.

We have followed closely the ancient progression set down centuries ago for practicing the Internal Energizing Exercises. One begins with the Deer, the Crane and the Turtle, and proceeds with the other exercises which work to heal the internal and external systems of the body. Once these initial exercises are mastered, one goes on to the meditative and breathing techniques. The special prescriptions for healing may be used whenever necessary. One may achieve proficiency and freedom from many previous weaknesses and diseases within three to six months after beginning to practice the initial exercises. Proficiency in the meditative and breathing techniques, however, may take from one to twenty years. Benefits accrue throughout the process however, and this allows us to observe their movement from time to time. We hope the growing sense of vitality and wellness which you feel upon following these exercises will be sufficient to keep you on the path toward physical, mental and spiritual enrichment.

THE DEER

The ancient Taoists understood that the human body could not exist unless there was a continual supply of energy coming into the tissues and organs. They realized that health was a condition which existed when the energy within the body was balanced — and that disease occurred when there was a state of energy depletion or weakness. We receive much of the energy we need from the food we eat and in the air we breathe. However, the body, much like an expensive automobile, must be finely tuned if it is to run properly and utilize this energy to its maximum level. Through the centuries, the seven glands within the body have been understood to be energy centers, responsible for regulating the flow of energy within the various systems in the body. The seven glands, in ascending order within the body, are: the sexual glands (male: prostate and testes; female: ovaries, uterus and mammary glands or breasts) which are responsible for hor-

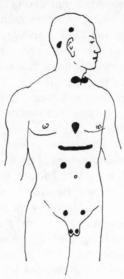

Fig. 1. Schematic Location of the Seven Glands.

mone secretions, sexual energy and response, and reproduction; the adrenals, which support the functioning of the kidneys, skin and spine; the pancreas, which helps maintain control over digestion, the blood sugar level and the heat of the body; the thymus, which governs the heart, lungs and the bones in the body; the thyroid gland, which maintains the metabolism of the cells in the body; the pituitary, which governs the mind, intelligence, memory, wisdom and thought; and the pineal gland, which directly affects the other glands through its secretions and rules over one's communication on a spiritual level.

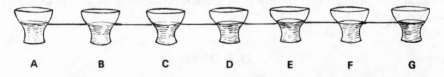

A   B   C   D   E   F   G

These seven glands may be visualized as vessels which are attached to one another by a series of arteries or tubes. Each vessel (gland) is dependent upon all the others for its supply of liquid (energy). If vessel A (the sexual glands) is supplied with liquid, this fluid will slowly disperse through the arteries to the remaining six vessels. Similarly, if vessel C (the pancreas) were to be drained excessively of its fluid (through a leak of some kind), each of the other vessels would give up a portion of their supply to reestablish an equilibrium within the system. This is similar to how energy flows within our bodies. A state of weakness or susceptibility to disease arises when one system, or in this case a gland, is for some

14

reason deprived of energy. Our task becomes then one of not only reestablishing the balanced flow of energy to overcome this weakness, but also to stimulate the flow of energy so that we raise the level of energy within our bodies to its maximum. Through this increase of energy we are then able to reverse our current weakness and heal ourselves, as well as to utilize the higher order of energy to open up our spiritual centers.

The sexual glands form the base of the glandular complex. The Chinese refer to these glands as the seven basic houses of the body. We need to understand that the seven glands support each other in an ascending order. If the first six glands are not filled to their capacity, then the seventh or spiritual house will not be filled either. We may quickly realize that if one were to surgically remove one of the glandular systems, there would be a permanent depletion or disequilibrium within the body. This is why, within the Chinese system of medicine, all available routes are explored before surgery is performed, especially if it involves the sexual glands (hysterectomy of prostectomy), as these comprise the basic or foundation house which supports all the rest. In such a case as removal of a gland, however, the Internal Exercises would still be important in providing a continued supply of energy to the body lest the person fall into a further weakened condition. On the other hand, one need not wait until all seven houses have been filled to capacity to experience benefits from the additional influx of energy which results from practicing the Internal Exercises. One may begin to feel within a few weeks the awakening or recharging of energy within the body and an accompanying decrease in disease symptoms or an increase in awareness, spiritual and/or psychic powers.

By exercising the rectum and anal muscles, one can strengthen, stimulate and energize the sexual glands. This simple action supplies energy to the thymus, which in turn pushes energy up into the succeeding glands which lie above it. This exercise is named after the deer, an animal which was observed to be continually stimulating its sexual glands by the movement of its tail from side to side throughout its life. The horns of the deer have been prized throughout antiquity as a powerful medicinal herb. The potency of the herb is believed to result from the deer's constant circulation of energy from its sexual glands, through its glandular system, and then into its head and horns. The horns, then, are actually a form of concentrated and highly powerful energy stored in a material form.

Taoists refer to the sexual glands as a stove, which when properly filled with wood and fire (stimulation and energy) supplies the rest of the house (body) with heat (energy). The Deer exercise, then, is a very basic and fundamentally important building block in the system of Internal Exercises. The exercise works to build up the sexual energy in the body. Often as a person experiences this increase in sexual energy, the tendency is to increase one's sexual exploits. Taoism allows for this possibility, but views promiscuity as a violation of the natural laws of healing. Anything, when carried to excess, leads to weakness or depletion of energy. On the other hand, leading a normal and active sexual life, while doing nothing to rebuild the lost energy which has been given up during sexual relations, is like burning a candle at both ends. One secret of continual youth is to maintain a reserve of energy by having strong sexual organs. This is one effect of the Deer exercise. (There is also a special treatise on the proper handling of the consequent increased sexual energy with respect to sexual relationships and intercourse.) It would be impossible to go into a lengthy discourse here. The authors' purpose herein is only to alert the practitioner to a possible pitfall in practicing this exercise and invites the reader to further research the Sexology of Taoism.

Another effect of the Deer is to strengthen the anal muscles and rectum. As one grows old and weak, one's anal opening tends to become very loose and flaccid. This is why many older persons, or those who have lost the use of the nerves which control the anus, through either paralysis or stroke, have a difficult time controlling their bowels. Anal muscles which have atrophied and become weak hasten the onset of diseases such as hemorrhoids and cancer. Thus one secret in maintaining youth into one's old age is to exercise these muscles and keep them strong.

In the male, the prostate lies behind the anal muscles. When the sphincter muscles are contracted, the prostate is exercised and strengthened. This helps prevent or even reverses many diseases associated with the prostate such as enlargement through overuse, or dysfunction through weakness and cancer. This is a boon to males over forty years of age who tend to suffer with problems of the prostate. In the female, when the anus is contracted, the vagina is exercised and strengthened. This stimulation helps cure and prevent such varied problems as colitis and vaginitis and other problems associated with the vagina and uterus.

The Deer is therefore a physical exercise as well as a mental and spiritual one. It improves one's sexual abilities as it builds up the energy reserves within the body. Fertility is increased and strengthened. Over time, the mental processes are heightened as well, and the outcome is often an increase in psychic powers and the growing feeling of an inner tranquility, which is a necessary prerequisite for the unfolding of one's spiritual centers.

THE MALE DEER EXERCISE

One may lie down on the side or back, sit or stand, whichever position is the most comfortable. (Please refer to Chapter Three, *Living with the Whole Body*, for information on the proper way to sit, lie and stand.) Begin by rubbing the palms of the hands together vigorously. This creates heat in the hands and brings the energy of the body into the palms and fingers. With the right hand, cup the testicles inside the hand so that the palm completely covers the scrotum. (The best way to perform this exercise is naked.) Do not squeeze; just a light pressure should be felt, as well as the heat from the hand going into the testicles. Place the palm of the left hand on the area of the pubis, one inch below the navel. Rotate the hand either clockwise or counterclockwise 81 times with a slight pressure so a gentle warmth begins to build in the area of the pubis. Then reverse the hands, making sure to rub the palms together vigorously to generate heat before starting again. Repeat the circular rubbing motion 81 times with the right hand on the pubis.

In Taoism, the number of Yang, or high, positive energy is nine. Hence, 9 x 9 = 81, or the highest possible Yang energy. So one rubs 81 times in this pose. When rubbing with the hands, concentrate with your full attention on an image of a growing fire within the sexual organs — the stove of the body. Keep your mind on the task. This form of concentration or Taoist meditation helps to increase the energy created by practicing the Deer exercise, and it helps unify the body and the mind, thus forming a whole and healthy unit.

After completing this part of the exercise with each hand, then tighten the muscles surrounding the anal opening. When done properly, it will feel as if air were being drawn up into the rectum. Tighten as hard as you can, and hold for as long as you comfortably are able. As with all Taoist exercises, you do not want to force the process. Forcing goes against the natural laws of healing and creates undue stress on the system. Perform the exercise until you are tired. Stop, then repeat it when you are rested. At first you may find you are only able to hold the sphincter muscles tight for several seconds. Please persist, and after several weeks, you will be able to hold the muscles tight for quite a while without experiencing tiredness or strain. When done properly, a pleasant feeling will be felt to travel from the base of the anus, through the spinal column, to the top of the head. This is due to pressure being placed on the prostate gland as it is gently massaged by the action of closing down the anal muscles. The sexual energy is thus diverted up the glandular system into the top of the head and to the pineal gland.

When you feel you have gained sufficient control over the anal muscles, then you may do the anal contraction while practicing the first part of the Deer exercise. This anal exercise may also be done independently of, or in conjunction with the other exercises, and is very important in strengthening the rectum and prostate. Among other things, this exercise cures and prevents hemorrhoids and cures problems of the prostate such as weakness, enlargement and cancer. It strengthens the nerve endings around the pubis and penis, and may be used to treat problems of impotence and premature ejaculation. Contraction of the anal muscles will also help enlarge the head or bulb of the penis, which will give the male more pleasant sensations during sexual intercourse.

It is crucial to learn control over the anal muscles if one is to master the later meditative and breathing Internal Exercises. These muscles may be visualized as a door or a lock. When shut, they close off the upper body and allow the energy to collect and build in the abdominal channel. Without this build-up of energy, it will be impossible to properly stimulate the sexual organs, and in turn, the other glands of the body. It is essential then to gain mastery over this lock if one is to strengthen one's system sufficiently to begin to energize the spiritual centers in the body.

Do this exercise in the morning upon rising and before retiring at night. (If the appropriate time is not available, once a day will have to suffice.) If an erection occurs while practicing this exercise, then place the

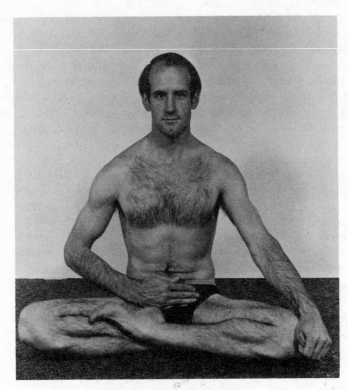

1. Deer Exercise (male).

thumb of the hand cupping the testicles at the base of the penis next to the pubis and press down sharply, while massaging the area of the pubis with the other hand. This will inhibit the flow of blood into the penis and maximize the build-up of energy within the sexual glands. (Taoist Sexology deals with the issue of proper orgasm without ejaculation to control the loss of energy during masturbation or sexual intercourse. The Teachings stress that one does not wish to experience ejaculation following this exercise, or at other times, except for purposes of procreation, as this dissipates the energy which has begun to build as a consequence of this exercise. Taoism stresses the proper use of sexual energy, not the suppression of sexuality.)

Proper hygiene must be practiced in conjunction with the Internal Exercises. We need to take the time daily to wash our entire bodies, including all the openings to the body. Social mores train us to wash the face, mouth and teeth thoroughly. We often neglect to wash the anal opening due to social taboos surrounding this particular area of the body. Please, take the time to clean the anal opening and the genitals so that germs and feces do not have a chance to collect, which can lead to infections, hemorrhoids or other weaknesses in this area of the body. Refer also to the Sun Worship and other exercises given in this book which work to energize the anal and genital areas of the body.

THE FEMALE DEER EXERCISE

Sit in a comfortable position on the floor or on a bed. Sit so that you can bring the heel of one foot so that it presses into and up against the opening of the vagina. You will want a steady and fairly hard pressure from the heel into the vagina, so that the heel presses tightly against the clitoris. If it is not possible to bring the foot into this position, then use a hard, round object such as a hard baseball to press against the vagina and clitoris. You may experience a pleasant sensation due to the stimulation of the genital area and a subsequent release of sexual energy. Begin by rubbing the hands together vigorously. This creates heat in the hands and brings the energy of the body into the palms and fingers. Place the hands on the breasts so that you feel the heat from the hands enter into the skin. Now rub with the hands in an outward, circular motion. (The right hand will turn in a counterclockwise manner; the left hand will turn in a clockwise motion.) Perform this circular motion a minimum of 36 times and a maximum of 306 times. At first your arms will become tired quite easily. But with patient practice, you will be able to perform this exercise comfortably. This outward circular rubbing motion of the hands is called *dispersion,* and helps to prevent or cure lumps and cancer of the breasts. One may reverse the motion of the hands to an inward rubbing motion. In this case the right hand circles in a clockwise fashion and the left hand rotates counterclockwise. This is called *stimulation* and its effect is to enlarge the breasts. When rubbing, always concentrate totally on the task. This form of concentration or meditation helps to unify the mind with the body and create a whole and healthy spiritual unit. As you perform this exercise, you will feel a warmth or fire building in the breasts and/or the genital region. This assures that the sexual energy is building within the body.

After finishing this part of the Deer exercise, then tighten the muscles of the vagina and anus as if you were trying to close both openings. When done properly, it will feel as if air were being drawn up into the rectum and vagina. Hold these muscles tight for as long as you comfortably can, then relax and repeat. You may feel a pleasant sensation rising from the genital area, up the spinal column and into the top of the head. This is caused by the build-up of sexual energy and its being directed up the glandular system into the head and pineal gland. As with all of the Taoist exercises, you do not want to force this action. This is and should be a natural rhythm. The first time you lock the anus, you may only be able to hold the muscles tight for a short time, but over time you will begin to build up the number of times you can do it, as well as the length of time you are able to hold the anal contractions.

When you are successfully able to control the anal muscles, you may perform this in conjunction with the hand rubbing. This anal/vaginal muscle contraction exercise may also be done independently of or in conjunction with all the other exercises.

The effects of this exercise are numerous and noteworthy. The exercise strengthens the muscles of the vagina and rectum and prevents and/or cures hemorrhoids. It cures and prevents vaginal problems such as infections, discharges, colitis, leucorrhea and menstrual disorders. It increases the circulation in the sexual organs and energizes the pubic area. It helps maintain youth and beauty by keeping the sexual glands (uterus, breasts and ovaries) strong and energized. It helps strengthen the energy in the body and creates an aura around the practitioner as well as helping to build up psychic ability.

Women are cautioned against performing the Deer during menstruation. At this time, a natural imbalance of hormones occurs within the body and this exercise may tend to further stimulate the imbalance. Women are also cautioned against performing the Deer exercise during pregnancy as the energy created by the exercise, and the accompanying increased stimulation of the glands, might induce premature labor.

Some women may find that their menstruation will stop as a result of practicing the Deer exercise. This is not a cause for alarm however, because the cessation of menstrual bleeding is a beneficial side effect of the Deer exercise. Now needless bleeding and the consequent loss of nutrition may be avoided and used instead to strengthen the female system and balance the organism. The normal menstrual cycle will return upon ceasing to perform the Deer exercise. There will be no detrimental side effects. The Taoists refer to this phenomenon as "turning back the blood" so that it may re-energize the entire body and especially the female sexual organs.

It is crucial to learn control over the anal muscles if one is to master the later meditative and internal breathing exercises. These muscles may be visualized as a door or a lock. In the female, as in the male, when shut, they close off the upper body and allow the energy to collect and build up

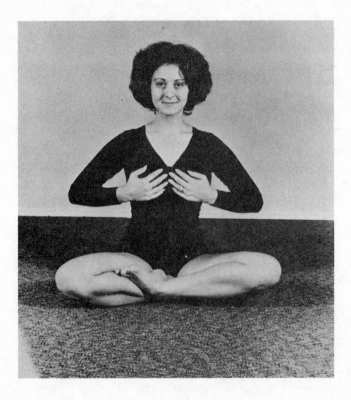

2. Deer Exercise (female).

in the abdominal channel. Without this build-up of energy, it is impossible to properly stimulate the sexual organs, and in turn, the other glands of the body. It is essential, then, to gain mastery over this lock if one is to strengthen one's system sufficiently to begin to energize the higher spiritual centers in the body.

Do this exercise in the morning upon rising and before retiring at night. If the appropriate time is not available, once a day will suffice. The same information in the previous section with regard to proper hygiene for men applies as well to women. The anus and genitals must be kept scrupulously clean and free from germs and feces. Refer also to the Sun Worship exercise and the other Internal Exercises which work to energize the anal and genital areas of the body.

PRONE POSITION FOR THE DEER EXERCISE

The prone position may be used as an alternative when one is unable to practice the Deer in a sitting position.

Begin by lying on your left side. (Since the Deer is performed for only a short period of time, one may lie on either the right or left side without straining the heart.) The left leg should be stretched straight out while the right leg, with the knee bent, lies on top. The left arm lies on the floor with the hand down toward the left leg, and the right arm is placed, with the hand down, in front of the body. Support the head with a cushion so the neck does not become strained. This position opens the pelvis so the anus and rectum may be contracted with ease. Perform the movements as outlined in the Deer exercise. (One may forego the hand rubbing on the pubis if this is too uncomfortable. The main benefit of the Deer is gained from the tightening of the anal muscles.)

Combine the breathing as taught in the Crane exercise to complete this pose. Repeat the breathing twelve times while simultaneously contracting the anal muscles. You may wish to practice this exercise while lying in the sunlight so that the sun bathes the anus and body in its health-enhancing and energy-producing light. Please refer ahead to Chapter Four for a complete description of the Sunlight Contemplation exercise.

THE CRANE

If one is to live a long and healthy life, it is necessary to have a strong internal system, including abdominal muscles, internal organs, lungs and circulatory system. The Crane is an exercise which was developed by the early Chinese Taoists to energize and strengthen these systems. The pose was appropriately named after the crane, a bird which appears to be constantly stimulating its abdominal area. As it stands, the crane will fold one leg into its belly, exerting pressure on its abdominal muscles and internal organs, which stimulates and strengthens its digestive, respiratory and circulatory systems.

Historically, as well as in modern times, man has suffered from many acute and chronic problems of the abdomen including constipation, diarrhea, ulcers, diverticulitis and cancers of the stomach, intestines and

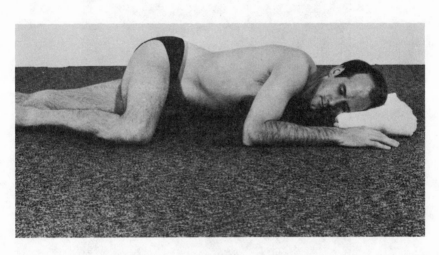

3. Prone Deer.

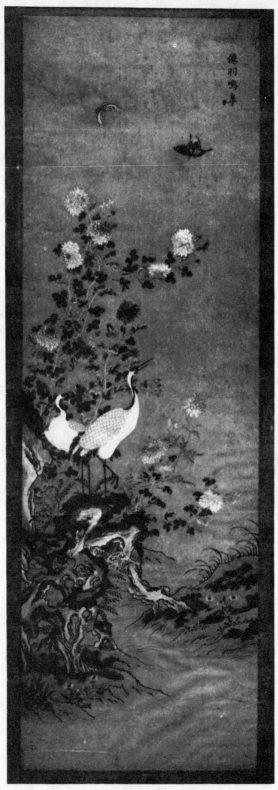

The Crane

colon. All of these diseases are caused by a similar problem — weakness in one or more parts of the digestive tract. When a tissue or an organ is weak, it is more susceptible to disease, and the greater the weakness, the more intense the symptoms. The digestive tract is controlled by the involuntary muscles. We need, then, to find a way to bring these muscles and organs under our control. We need to force the stomach, intestines and colon to move, to work so they may be strengthened. Normally, when we breathe, the lungs tend to expand outward toward the chest. The Crane exercise, however, forces the lungs downward and because the intestines have nowhere to go, they are pressed outward against the abdominal muscles to form a little ball. This motion breaks up constipation, encourages absorption of nutrition, and strengthens the entire digestive tract while stimulating the lungs and circulatory system. In this way, invading germs do not have a good environment in which to settle and germinate because one's bowel movements are so strong and regular. Then it is not easy to get disease. The Crane also increases the circulation to the abdominal organs and muscles and reduces the accumulation of cholesterols and fats in the blood stream. The pose helps cure asthma through its effects on the lungs, and because the lungs and skin work together as a unit, the pose helps to cure skin disorders such as rashes and sores.

Poor breathing habits are a major cause of weakness and disease in the body. One tends to breathe using only the upper half of the lungs and only rarely does one utilize the lower portion of the lungs. During a typical day, we exchange about one pint of air with each breath. Were we to breathe deeper, we would take in an additional three pints of air. Even on a full inhalation, we could add only another three pints of air. This would still leave a residual of three pints of air in the lungs. One quickly realizes that because of our daily shallow breathing habits, we receive one tenth of our total lung capacity of air with each breath. Problems such as headache, indigestion and dizziness come from lack of oxygen in the blood. Poor circulation, a problem of old age, and unfortunately, a problem which more and more young people are suffering from as well, comes from these improper breathing patterns.

The air we breathe contains oxygen, nitrogen, carbon and other trace elements which we need for our survival. The air we breathe also contains energy, without which we could not survive. This energy is called *Chi* (Qi): It is the vital energy of the body. We can now understand why it is crucial for our survival to develop proper breathing habits, for we depend on the air we breathe to give us not only oxygen, which is the fuel our bodies run on, but to provide us with *energy*, which is the spark of life, without which we would quickly grow weak and die. We want, therefore, to exercise the lower lungs. For this reason, we should follow the example of the crane. This is a very basic foundation exercise in the system of Taoist Internal Exercises. The breathing, as taught in the Crane, is also the basis for future meditative and advanced breathing techniques which will be presented later.

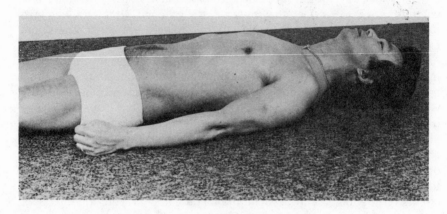

4. Crane Breathing Exercise (1).

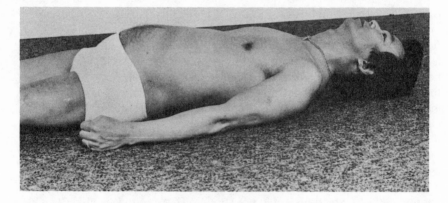

5. Crane Breathing Exercise (2).

26

THE CRANE EXERCISE

This pose may be practiced while standing, sitting or while assuming a prone position. Begin by rubbing the palms of the hands together vigorously. Once again, this creates heat in the hands and brings the energy of the body into the palms and fingers. Then place the hands, palms down, on the lower abdomen so that they lie on either side of the navel. Now begin to exhale slowly, and at the same time press the hands down lightly so that the abdomen forms a hollow cavity. This motion forces the air out of the abdomen and lower lungs. In this instance, the hands are like the leg of the crane. We want to imagine that every drop of air is leaving the lungs. After you exhale completely, begin to inhale slowly, and extend the abdomen outward so that it becomes like a balloon. Try not to allow the chest to expand — you want to use only the muscles in the lower abdomen while doing the Crane breathing. It is not necessary to force either the inhale or the exhale. With continued practice, you will be able to extend and empty the abdomen quite easily while breathing very slowly. You do want to center your entire concentration on the area surrounding the navel and imagine that you are only using your lower lungs with which to breathe. In the beginning, the hands act as guides to help you to learn the pose. Once mastered, however, the pose does not require the use of the hands on the abdomen. One complete exhale followed by an inhale comprises one round of breathing.

Once you have mastered the breathing technique, you may perform the anal lock as described in the Deer exercise with the breathing, by tightening the muscles around the anus. This will increase the strength of the pose and also tends to increase the energy created by performing the Crane as well as the benefits one derives from it.

The best time to do the Crane breathing is in the morning, and if possible, while facing the sun. The sun represents life and positive energy, and we want to bring as much of this life as we can into our bodies. Imagine that as you inhale, you are bringing this vital energy into the body, filling it up completely. As you exhale, imagine that all the toxins and wastes from the body are leaving. At first, you will only be able to perform two or three rounds of breathing at one sitting. Eventually you want to perform twelve repetitions when practicing the Crane. Always remember to breathe slowly. You may also wish to do the Crane before retiring at night. The position gives a gentle massage to the inner organs which helps calm the body, a necessary requisite for proper sleep.

Women are cautioned not to perform the Crane during pregnancy as the in/out motions of the abdomen may create unpleasant feelings within the abdomen.

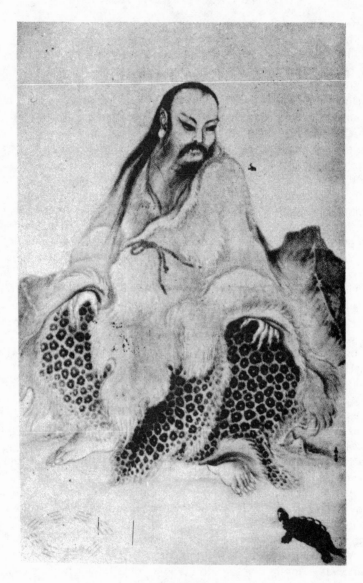

The Turtle

THE TURTLE

Ancient Taoist texts tell the story of a family which escaped to the hills during a time of war. They took up residence in a cave deep within the mountains. One day, a large boulder crashed down, sealing the family within the cave. No amount of digging from inside could free them, so they sat to await the chance that someone would discover their plight. Months passed, and the family anxiously awaited their death due to their dwindling supply of food. One day, they discovered a turtle which had been in the cave with them from the beginning. The turtle had been so still that they had earlier mistaken it for a rock. Now they studied it with the utmost fascination, wondering how it had been able to survive until now. As they observed it over the following days, they found the only movements it made were to extend and shrink its head in and out of its shell. Occasionally, it would stop to catch on its tongue a drop of water which had fallen from the ceiling. It had no other sustenance. Soon the family was out of food. Facing starvation, with nothing else to guide them, they began to imitate the movements of the turtle in hopes the simple exercise would somehow keep them alive. Many years passed before others discovered the family and removed the boulder which had blocked their escape. When the records were checked, it was found that 800 years had passed since the time the family had first been locked in the cave! News of their survival soon spread and their fellow countrymen were astonished on learning that only a few drops of water and a simple exercise imitating the movements of a tortoise had sustained them through the centuries.

You may not believe this story, and we recite it only to encourage people to follow the Turtle exercise, but the Turtle pose is one which stimulates the nerves. It stretches, stimulates and energizes all the nerves of the neck which lead to the brain and to the lower extremities of the body. The neck forms the central pathway for all the nerves leading to and from the brain through the central nervous system. If we are able to gain control over this complex of nerves, then we control the entire functioning of the body. We can cut off an arm and remain alive. However, if our head were to be cut off, death would follow instantly. One must recognize the importance of exercising this area, as it increases the circulation and carries away deposits which would otherwise impair the proper functioning of the nerves, tissues, arteries and veins of the neck.

The Turtle stretches the entire spine, energizes the neck, strengthens the shoulder muscles and removes stiffness, soreness and tiredness from the neck and shoulder muscles. In addition, the thyroid and parathyroid glands are stimulated and strengthened, improving the body's metabolism. If one performs the Turtle on a daily basis, one will feel younger and radiate an inner beauty which comes only through the proper functioning of one's inner energy systems.

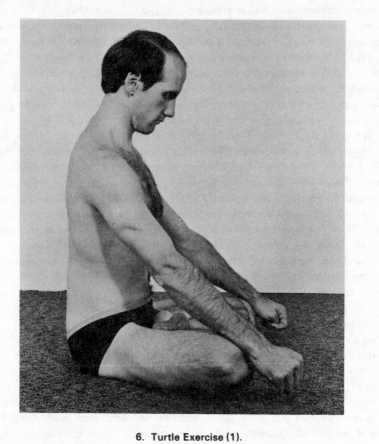

6. Turtle Exercise (1).

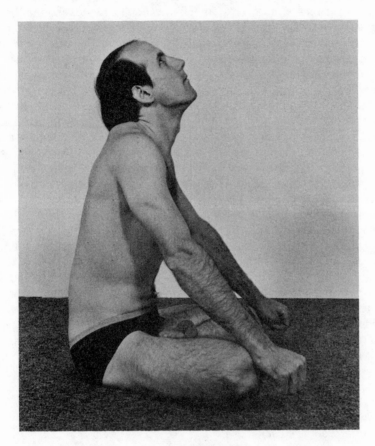

7. Turtle Exercise (2).

THE TURTLE EXERCISE

Sit or stand in a comfortable position. (In cases of persons who are bedridden, the exercise may be performed lying down. Also, please consult the positions for standing and sitting properly in Chapter Three.) Begin by bringing the chin down into the chest and stretching the top of the head upward. The back of the neck will feel a stretch upward and the shoulders will relax downward. Then slowly bring the back of the skull down as if to touch it on the back of the neck. The chin will pull upward, and the throat will be slightly stretched. The shoulders will now pull upward on either side of the head as if you were trying to touch them to the ears. These two movements mimic the tortoise, from which the exercise derives its name, as the animal pulls its head in and out of its shell. None of the movements need be forced, and you may find it helpful to synchronize the movements of the Turtle with the breathing you learned in the Crane pose. In this case, as you stretch the head upward, inhale; as you bring the head down and the chin up, exhale. In any case, please proceed slowly, with natural movements. Understand that it may take a number of attempts before you feel comfortable practicing this exercise. Patience in practicing this exercise will lead you to a treasure of medical, emotional, and spiritual benefits. Upon performing the pose correctly, you may immediately feel a diminishing of any tension or tiredness in the neck or upper back.

You will want to do the Turtle twelve repetitions each time you practice it. The best time to perform the exercise is in the early morning upon rising, and just before retiring at night. It may also be practiced any time you feel tension or tightness in the neck or upper back and shoulders. While doing the Turtle, look straight ahead with soft or muted light, or keep the eyes gently closed. You want to hold the rest of the body relaxed and keep the fingers clasped around the thumbs as you make a fist. This is a hand lock and prevents any energy from spilling out through the hands. Always remember to concentrate on what you are doing. If the mind wanders, bring it gently back. By concentrating all your thoughts on the movements made by the body while practicing the Turtle, you increase the benefits derived from doing the position and help unify the mind and the body. This is an important concept to keep in mind as you perform all of the Internal Energizing Exercises.

COMBINING THE THREE FOUNDATION EXERCISES

Once one is able to comfortably practice the three foundation exercises on an individual basis, then the Deer, Crane and Turtle may be put together and performed as one basic exercise. This is accomplished by combining the component parts of each exercise into one single exercise. Basically, one will synchronize the neck stretching as learned in the Turtle, with the breathing as taught in the Crane, together with the anal lock and hand rubbing as taught in the Deer (eventually the hand rubbing may be discontinued and only the anal lock used). This may seem a bit confusing when first practiced, but if one has become proficient in the individual exercises before putting them together, it should not take long to master this combination technique.

Each of the three exercises, as well as the combination technique when mastered, should be practiced daily, preferably once in the morning and again at night for optimum benefits. If one were only to practice these three basic exercises, one's health would expand a great deal. The Crane will strengthen and stimulate the circulatory and digestive systems. If these two complexes are strong, then it will not be easy to accumulate weakness and disease. The Deer stimulates the physical as well as the spiritual being of the practitioner. It improves one's sexual energy and insures a balanced glandular and hormonal system. It is said that if one has strong sexual glands, one may never grow old. The Turtle energizes the nerves and strengthens the brain, spinal column and neck region. Possessing a strong central nervous system helps balance one's mental energy and eventually helps to bring peace of mind.

The Taoist teachings are very practical. They teach that we are each responsible for our own state of being — physical, mental and emotional, as well as spiritual. One is asked to follow the exercises on a daily basis. Do the exercises one day at a time. This is a step-by-step process. One need not be in a rush to get somewhere, as the process is one of unfolding, and that can never be hurried. One need only take the time and possess the interest to continue with the exercises. In time, you will gain the ability to travel within your own body and heal yourself. By bringing the physical and mental bodies into harmony, one provides fertile ground for the spontaneous growth of intelligence and a strong spiritual state of being. This is the main emphasis of all the Taoist teachings.

3 Living with the Whole Body

In addition to the three foundation exercises, Taoist teachings offer correct methods for sitting, standing, lying down and walking. People tend to sacrifice much of their everyday energy in supporting unhealthy forms of posture. These suggestions, as recorded here, provide simple ways of arranging our bodies so that we enhance rather than retard the natural flow of energy as we go about our daily lives. A number of additional exercises are also recommended, the purpose of which is to stimulate, energize and strengthen all the organs, tissues and cells in the body. In Chinese medicine, every doctor knows that the eyes are the opening to the liver. If the liver doesn't function properly, you are going to develop eye problems. Similarly, if there are problems with the eyes, one looks to the liver for the source of the problem. The nose is the pathway to the lungs. Allergies indicate that the lungs may not be functioning properly. The ears are the opening to the kidneys and the mouth is the opening to the stomach. One needs, then, individual exercises which will stimulate these and other areas of the body to keep them functioning properly.

The proper use of thought, imagination and visualization plays an important part in each of the Internal Exercises. It has been recognized for centuries that a thought is as much a reality as a material object, and in fact, that they are one and the same. They are both forms of energy, the distinguishing difference being that they exist at different frequencies and wave lengths of vibration. Imagination and visualization are used, then, to bring together the mind and the body so that they function as a unit. Spontaneity is the total harmonization of mind and body. By visualizing a flow of energy, we may begin to set the stage for our becoming aware of the actual flow of energy which, in the beginning, may be occurring at levels "below" our ordinary consciousness. By using our imagination, we may begin to explore our minds and bodies through the Internal Exercises, and in time we will discover extraordinary vistas and levels of health existing within us.

Belief in the Internal Exercises is not necessary for them to work. Realize, however, that negative thoughts can and often do lead to states of malfunctioning and disease. One needs to cultivate an open mind, much like that of a child; then we may experience the efficacy of these simple exercises for ourselves and come to know the truths which they contain.

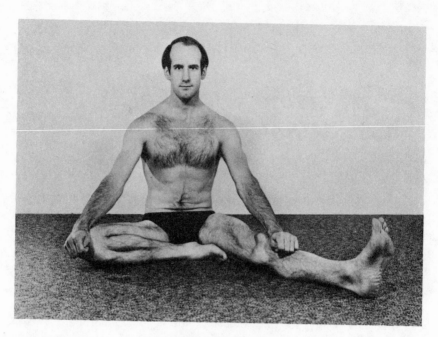

8. Sitting Position (1).

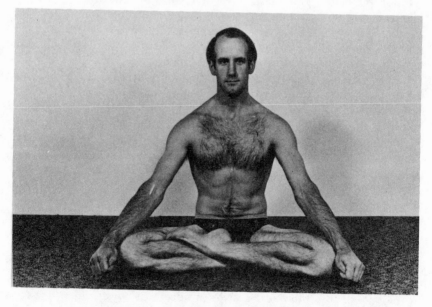

9. Sitting Position (2).

THE SITTING POSITION

Sitting correctly increases one's energy and improves the health of the body even as one sits. It is best to sit with the heel of one foot pressed tightly against the perineum. For the male, the heel will press against the prostate; for the female, the heel will press against the clitoris. The other leg may be kept extended or brought upon the opposite leg to form the half lotus position. If neither of these postures is comfortable, one may use an object such as a hard ball to put pressure on the prostate or clitoris as one sits. Remember to always keep the spine as straight as possible. One may also practice locking the sphincter muscles around the anus while in this position, but understand that keeping the anus locked all the time will result in too much tension in the body, causing a negative reaction. One needs to observe moderation in all these exercises. There need never be strain or overexertion to obtain the maximum benefits from the Internal Exercises.

This sitting position opens the pelvis so that the heel may be pressed comfortably into the perineum. Through overuse of the sexual organs, we lose a great deal of energy. Even through inactivity the sexual organs may grow weak. Since the sexual organs are the basic gland in the body, they need to be protected and energized. This sitting position protects against the loss of energy through the "gate of heaven," or prostate and clitoris, and enables one to build up additional energy in the sexual glands.

When sitting on a chair or on a couch, keep the thighs parallel to the floor, with the spine erect. This is the healthiest position for regular sitting. One does not want a chair to be so high that the feet have difficulty touching the ground, nor so low that the knees are above the thighs. Sitting back in a plush sofa may seem comfortable at first, but it promotes poor posture and is not a healthy way to sit. The bones do not align properly, the vertebrae become crooked and one's energy does not flow correctly through the spinal column. The two methods for correct sitting described here are to be used whenever one practices the Internal Exercises — including the breathing and meditation techniques — as well as when one works at a desk, listens to another, or is simply reading a book. Sitting properly promotes a healthy flow of energy in the body and keeps the mind in an alert and responsive state.

THE STANDING POSITION

When standing, keep the feet shoulder width apart and parallel to each other. One's weight should be evenly distributed along the feet. Too much weight on the heels throws the spine off center, makes the abdomen sag, stimulates too many nerves in the heel, and makes the brain lazy. If anything, keep the weight forward toward the ball of the foot. This keeps the mind alert and gives one a feeling of lightness in the body.

THE STANDING CRANE

This exercise is similar to the sitting Crane exercise, only it is per-

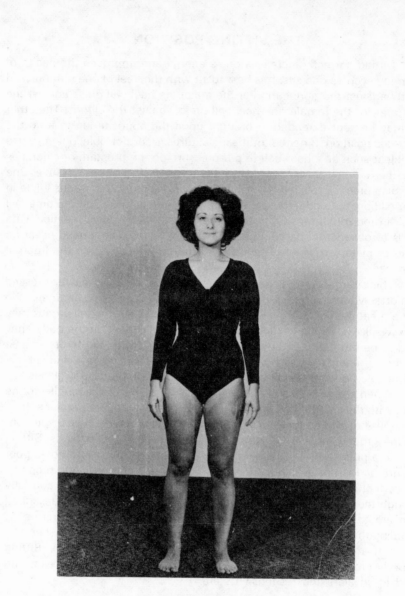

10. Standing Pose (alternative).

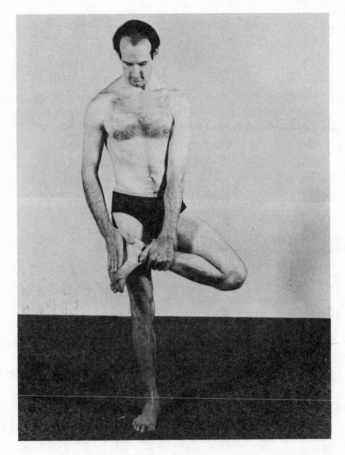

11. Standing Crane (1).

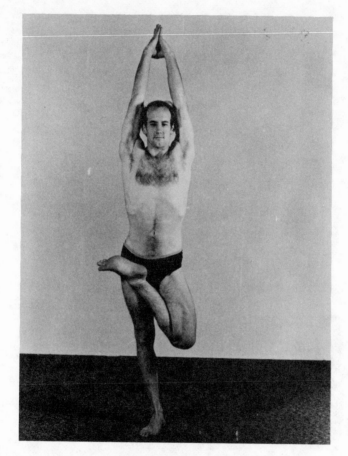

12. Standing Crane (2).

formed while standing. It helps develop balance, stimulates the nervous system, strengthens the inner organs and increases the flexibility of the knee, ankle and hip joints. It increases the circulation in the legs and feet and reverses tendencies toward cramps in the legs and feet, varicose veins and cold feet.

Assume a standing position with the feet together, toes and heels touching. Pick up one foot and begin by rubbing the sole of the foot on the opposite foreleg. Gradually work the foot up the leg, stopping every few inches or so to continue the rubbing motion, until the foot rests on the outside thigh of the opposite leg. The heel will be in toward the pelvis and the toes will extend past the thigh near the hip joint. Now massage the sole of the foot with the hands and manipulate the toes to stimulate the nerves and circulation in the foot. Next, slowly raise the arms over the head sideways as you inhale and bring the palms as close together as possible. Breathing normally, try to balance in this position for as long as you feel comfortable. Then, upon exhalation, lower the arms and repeat with the other foot.

It may not be possible to balance in the full position at first, but with continued practice the pose will open up and you will find yourself performing it with ease. The increased ability to balance will have enormous beneficial effects on your everyday life.

WALKING

When walking, never hurry, lest you build up an excessive amount of tension and make the heart beat too rapidly. It is better not to run unless necessary. Leave early for your destination and avoid needless stress and tension; stress is perhaps the biggest enemy of the body. When one gets going too fast, there is a build-up of unnecessary tension. Over a period of time, this may lead to weakness and to diseases such as cancer and ulcers.

While walking, one's steps should be even, and only the legs should be used so that the mind remains alert and peaceful. Always walk with complete attention to and awareness of what you are doing. Walk at a constant speed, not too fast or too slow, but at just an easy gait. The feet should remain parallel, with the heels and toes pointing straight ahead. When you walk correctly, you will feel like a cloud: Balanced, light and airy.

BONE BREATHING FOR COMPLETE RELAXATION

We need a certain amount of tension to live, as the total absence of tension is death. However, it is a medical fact that excessive tension and stress cause disease, quite probably even cancer. Taoists have understood for centuries that the best way to protect against disease is to give oneself a full body-and-mind relaxation at least once a day. Relaxation is of the utmost importance for proper healing to take place as it helps prevent energy blocks caused by the build-up of tension.

Begin by lying on the back with the feet slightly apart, the arms next to the body with the palms slightly upturned. Allow the floor or bed to sup-

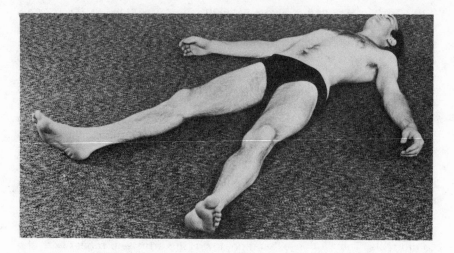

13. Bone Breathing — complete relaxation.

port the weight of the body rather than using your muscles to hold you up off the floor. Keep the eyes closed and let the breathing become regular. As you inhale, imagine that fresh, clean air, energy and vitality are entering into and penetrating throughout your body. As you exhale, imagine that all the toxins and stale air are leaving the body. Do not underestimate the power of your imagination. Ideas are as much a reality as is the table which has been built from them.

Now begin to imagine that as you inhale, the air comes in through the toes and up through the bones of the leg and enters into your chest. As you breathe out, imagine the air descending through the chest, passing through the leg and out through the toes of the foot. Repeat this movement three times with each leg. Then imagine that the air comes up through the hands and arms, entering into the chest and head. On the exhale, follow the air back down through the arm and out through the hand. Repeat this movement three times with each arm. Once you have mastered the individual movements, you may combine the flow of the breath through both the arms and legs simultaneously.

Upon completing the Bone Breathing exercise, your mind and body will feel completely rested and relaxed and you will feel refreshed and ready to begin your work anew. If it is not practical to assume a prone position (for example, when you are at work or are traveling on a bus or plane), then close your eyes and practice the exercise in a sitting position with the spine as straight as possible and the arms and legs in a relaxed and comfortable position.

SLEEPING

The best position for sleeping is lying on the back. Many people experience nightmares when first assuming this sleeping position — however, the nightmares should disappear after a little while. The next best position is to lie on your right side. If you lie on your left side, the lungs, stomach and liver will press onto your heart; this additional weight strains the heart and may be a factor in causing heart disease. Avoid sleeping on your stomach. This puts an excessive amount of pressure on the lungs, heart and internal organs, produces shallow breathing habits, and often results in severe neck strain and pain due to the head and neck being twisted.

Try to sleep in a well-ventilated room, preferably with your head to the north and your feet to the south so you are in line with the natural flow of energy in the universe. Avoid oversleeping. This makes the body sluggish and promotes weakness, as does too little sleep. Between seven and eight hours of sleep is sufficient for the average person. If you need more than that, it may be that your system has become weakened through improper exercise, diet or living habits.

TOE WIGGLING AND BODY STRETCHING

During sleep, or for that matter during any prolonged period of inactivity, toxins accumulate in the muscles due to the decrease in circulation which results in stiffness. Old age is often said to begin in the toes, as older people often suffer from poor circulation and cold feet. What we need then is to stretch the body upon rising to help break up the toxins and restore the proper circulation to the muscles and tissues in the body. This helps us to wake up and become alert more quickly. If you observe animals such as the cat, you will see that when they wake up, the first thing they do is stretch their bodies. They are following a natural law which we too need to follow. So, upon rising in the morning, and while still in bed, stretch your arms, legs, back and feet. It does not matter which way — just stretch. Be very free about it, following no particular form or style. After you stretch, pause briefly to relax before getting up.

Now you need to move and stimulate the toes. Wiggle the big toes back and forth several times. By moving the large toe, you stimulate all the nerves in the body. All the systems of the body are reflected in the nerve endings on the feet. This is coincident to the science currently known as reflexology. The related sciences of reflexology and zone therapy have been known and practiced for over 6,000 years. When one wiggles the toes, the liver is exercised and stimulated, and energy is sent to the sexual glands. By doing this exercise, you will have at one stroke stimulated the whole body through the feet. Wiggle the toes twelve times. Make sure that you closely attend to the movements of the toes, so that the exercise becomes a mediation as well. This will increase the benefit you derive from this exercise.

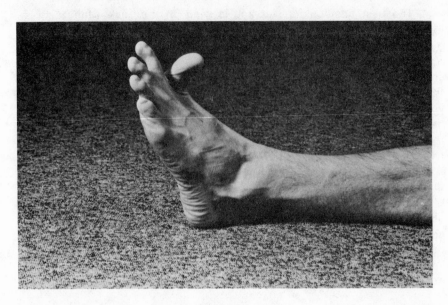

14. Toe Wiggling (1).

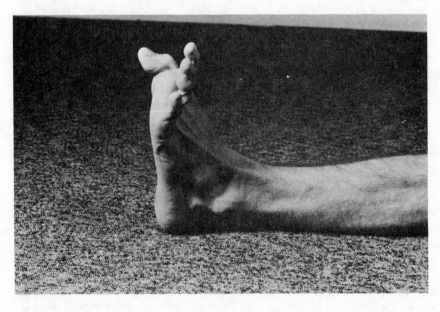

15. Toe Wiggling (2).

HEAD RUBBING
Part One

Press hands on head points as indicated in the accompanying photo. Do not scratch these points, simply rub back and forth on the skin without removing the hands from the head. This is an excellent exercise for stimulating the circulation in the scalp and to stop the hair from falling out because the hair follicles become nourished with the added circulation.

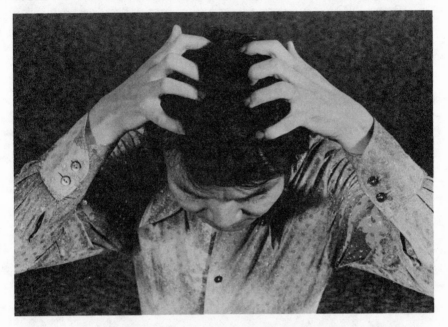

16. Head Rubbing—beauty and fitness.

Part Two

Press the fingers into the points on the back of the neck to help remove tension and fatigue from the upper back and neck. Press in and rub at the same time. This wonderful exercise helps eliminate tension headaches on a preventive basis by preventing tension from building in the neck. It is also an excellent tonic when you have a headache and wish to get rid of it.

Fig. 2.

Head Rubbing—Part Two.

INTERNAL ORGAN RELAXATION

The internal organs of four-legged animals hang freely within the abdomen, and so they are always assured the proper amount of blood. The organs of a human being, however, are piled one on top of the other when standing erect. We need, then, to give these organs a chance to relax and have some free space so that they might enjoy proper circulation. Once again, we need to follow the example given to us by other animals.

Begin this in the morning after stretching the body and exercising the toes. Roll over on your bed or onto the floor so that the toes, legs, knees and hands are on the floor. You will be like a dog, with the head for-

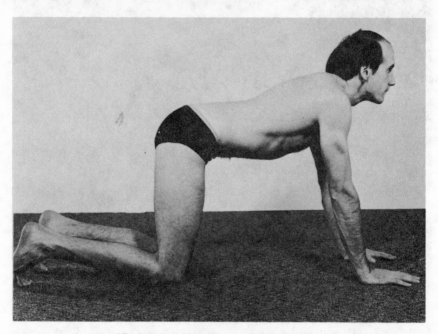

17. Internal Organ Relaxation (alternative).

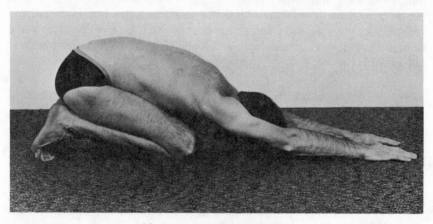

18. Internal Organ Relaxation.

46

ward and the chest parallel to the floor. Pause a moment to allow blood to circulate freely into and around all the internal organs. Then slowly sit back on your heels and lower your forehead toward the floor. The arms will stretch out in front of you. Close the eyes and remain in this position for a few seconds, then come back to the kneeling position. You may want to synchronize your breathing with the movements of the exercise, but however you do it, always keep the breathing easy and natural. Repeat the exercise seven times.

In this exercise, blood is retained in the stomach and the intestines, which strengthens digestion and elimination. Sitting down onto the heels forces blood to flow to the heart, lungs and brain. Blood then flows back to the heart easily so that the heart has a chance to rest. During a sound sleep, the flow of blood is reduced to the head. We need to start with this pose in the morning to bring the blood to our brain so that we will feel fresh, alert and alive.

Those who have high blood pressure are cautioned not to practice this position until their blood pressure has been brought to within normal limits through the practice of the other internal exercises. (Please see prescriptions to be performed in cases of high blood pressure.) This pose tends to bring too much blood to the brain and increases one's blood pressure, so that it may be dangerous for persons suffering from high blood pressure to perform this exercise. It would also be wise for the average person to work into this pose gradually. One does not want to put such pressure on the brain too quickly. Allow the arteries, veins and capillaries to accommodate over time to the increased flow of blood caused by this exercise. At first, practice the pose once or twice, slowly working up to seven times over a period of a few weeks.

HEALING AND STRENGTHENING THE EYES

The eyes are the opening to the liver. Chinese medicine explains that persons suffering from eye problems suffer from disorders in their liver. Conversely, persons who have a liver problem will eventually develop eye problems. Through proper stimulation of the eyes and the surrounding area, we can strengthen both the eyes and liver and cure many so-called irreversible disorders such as cataract, astigmatism, nearsightedness, glaucoma, and problems of the liver. Eye movements are also indicative of a person's intelligence. People who are clever have large eye movements and are always exploring their environment. Slow eye movement or a lack of eye movement indicates a repressed level of intelligence, which may also be helped through stimulation of the eyes.

There are meridian points which lie along the bones surrounding the eyes. These points or openings to the pathways of energy which supply the eyes need to be exercised to stimulate the energy flow and break up blocks in the energy flow which may occur from time to time through eye strain, overexertion or exposure to poor environmental conditions such as air pollution. Begin by pressing point A on each eye with the thumbs. Exert heavy pressure upon the points. If you feel any pain, even with a very intense pressure, this means that there is a weakness in the eyes. When the

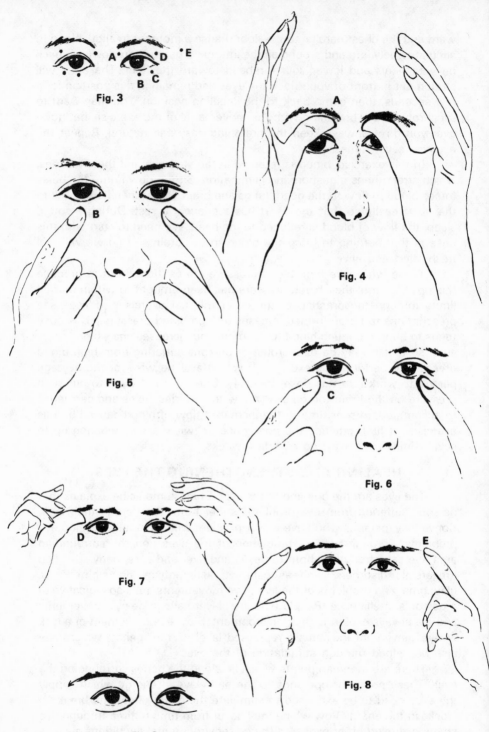

Fig. 3

Fig. 4

Fig. 5

Fig. 6

Fig. 7

Fig. 8

Fig. 9

Figs. 3.-9.   Eye Exercises.

eyes are in a healthy state, there will be an absence of all pain. Press in deeply for about ten seconds. Then rub the points with the thumbs, again using strong pressure. Next, press each of the succeeding points B, C, D, E, and F, using the fingers and following each pressing with the rubbing motion. Completion of all five points forms one round of this exercise. Repeat for a total of three rounds. Then, using the fingers, rub the bones around the eyes in a circular motion starting from the inside of each eye near the nose and rubbing up the bridge of the nose and across the eyebrows toward the temples and back around. This rubbing sends additional energy into the eyes and helps to reduce wrinkles of the skin around the eyes. (One does not want to rub in the opposite direction for this will tend to weaken the eye muscles and cause wrinkles to appear.) Rub for several seconds, then rub the palms of the hands together vigorously. Place the palms over the eyes and feel the warmth enter into the eyes.

If one suffers from severe eye problems such as cataract or glaucoma, practice this exercise up to twenty minutes daily until the problem abates. Otherwise, a few minutes' attention to this exercise daily will help keep the eyes in a healthy state. You may find that problems such as nearsightedness will slowly disappear and that the vision will become very sharp and clear. Whenever the eyes become tired, stop what you are doing and practice this exercise. It is helpful to do this in the morning after performing the Internal Organ Relaxation. The exercise which strengthens the liver should also be done in conjunction with this exercise.

To cure difficult eye problems, or merely to keep the eyes healthy, one may also practice additional exercises that will strengthen the eyes and the muscles surrounding them. Examine the diagram and begin by

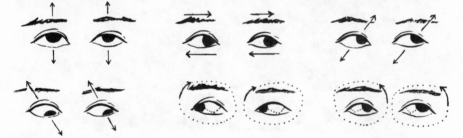

Fig. 10. Eye Motions.

keeping the head straight, but with the eyes first looking up toward the ceiling and then down at the floor. Repeat this motion several times. The eyes should always move slowly and with deliberation. Next, look to either side of the head. Then look up and down into the opposite corners of the eyes. Rotate the eyes first in a clockwise direction, then in a counterclockwise direction. This will take about ten minutes to perform when done slowly. Always follow these eye movements with rubbing of the hands and pressing the palms onto the eyes to bring heat and energy into them. If you practice these exercises consistently over a period of time, you will never need to see an eye doctor again and you may eventually throw your glasses away.

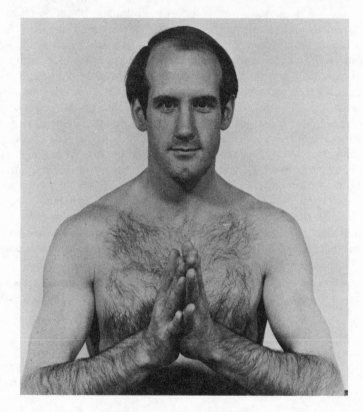

19. Eye Exercise — Palming (1).

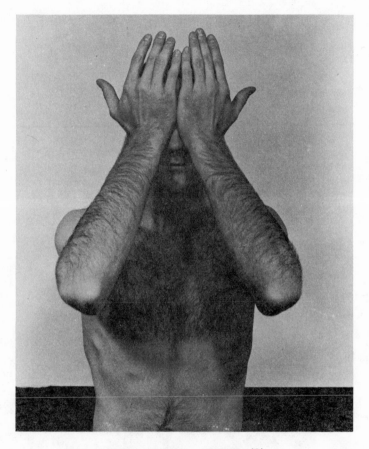

20. Eye Exercise — Palming (2).

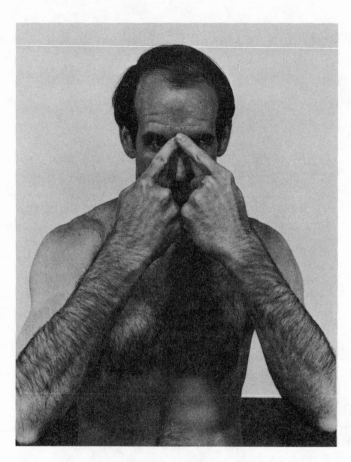

21. Nose Exercise (1).

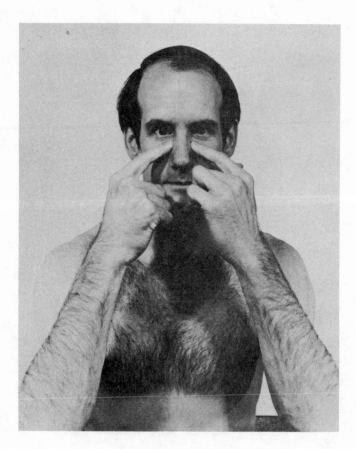

22. Nose Exercise (2).

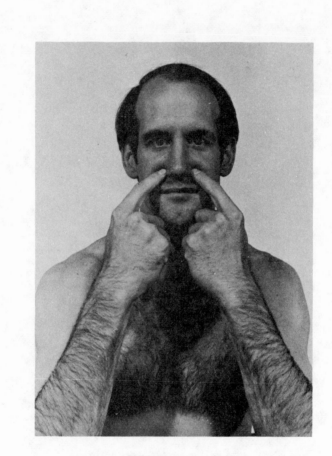

23. Nose Exercise (3).

THE NOSE, LUNGS AND SINUSES EXERCISE

The nose is the opening to the lungs. Symptoms such as allergy, runny nose and blocked sinuses are the manifestations of weakness within the lungs. To strengthen the lungs one needs to perform the Crane exercise, which directs a flow of energy that helps restore any degenerative conditions within the pulmonary system. We can also help keep the lungs strong, as well as keep the sinuses healthy, by stimulating certain points around the nose. These are spots which open up into the meridians which supply the nose and surrounding areas with energy. By pressing these points, we insure a continual flow of energy through the nasal and sinus passages.

Using the tip of the index or the second fingers of each hand, press down with heavy pressure on the three points as indicated in the diagram. Begin at the base of the nose and press this point for about ten seconds. Then rub the fingers on these two spots and proceed to press the points midway up on either side of the nose. Press, then rub with a steady pressure. Then press the point midway between the eyebrows (the third eye) with both fingers. Repeat this progression three times, always beginning with the lower points and ending by pressing the point corresponding to the third eye. Next, rub in a continual flowing motion, starting at the lowest point, passing through the second and third points and then continuing up through the middle of the forehead. Repeat this movement three times. Throughout the exercise, the pressure exerted should be penetrating and deep. Often when just beginning, the points will be sensitive or slightly painful. This is an indication of weakness or a blockage within the meridian. Continue to perform this exercise daily and the pain will disappear in time. You may notice that you will acquire fewer colds, allergy and sinus conditions.

Practice this exercise in the morning after performing the eye exercises. Then you may repeat this pose as many times during the day as you feel are necessary to help with your sinus or nasal problems. If you find yourself in a heavily polluted atmosphere, such as a construction site, you may wish to do this exercise to help flush out the dirt and stimulate your nose.

BEATING THE HEAVENLY DRUM

Whether it be daytime or nighttime, one's environment never rests. When you are sleeping you may think you hear nothing, but the ears are still receiving stimuli. If someone were to drop a heavy object next to you, you would quickly awaken. The Taoist teachings, however, show a way to rest the ears. They call this exercise "Beating the Heavenly Drum."

Place the index fingers of each hand on the outside of the ears and fold over the outside flaps of skin which lie next to the opening to the inner ear canal so that you seal off the ear from the outside. Using the tips of the second fingers, tap gently on the fingernails of the index fingers. When done properly, you will hear a metallic sound much like the beating of a drum. You must tap a regular rhythm, slowly, twelve to thirty-six times. Then pause, and repeat for a total of three times.

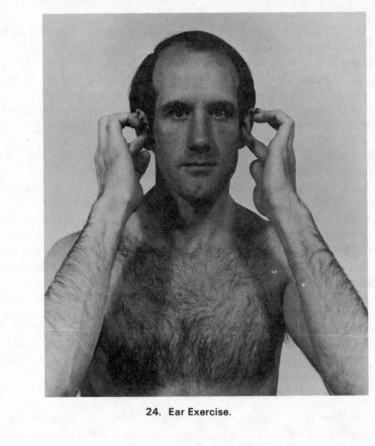

24. Ear Exercise.

When you first close off the ears, before you begin tapping, you will hear a sound much like that made by a waterfall. The ear is still working! After following this exercise for a few days, the sound of the waterfall will cease after doing the exercise, and will be replaced by a calm silence. This exercise stimulates and gives rest to the inner ear. It is very important to keep the ears healthy, and by following this exercise, you will insure yourself good hearing into old age. Many diseases of the ears, such as ringing and partial deafness, can be helped or cured by using this exercise.

In Chinese medicine, the ears are regarded as the opening to the kidneys. So if you do have problems with your ears, it is a warning signal that you have a weakness in your kidneys. It is important then to also practice the kidney stimulating exercise along with the ear exercise.

The ears lie in line with, and are connected to, the pineal gland, which, as you may recall, is the center for spiritual awareness. Practicing the ear exercise stimulates the pineal gland and helps to keep it healthy and energized. You may find you feel very tranquil after performing this exercise.

Practice the ear stimulating exercise in the morning after working on the nose. Then you may perform it as often as you like during the day. Those who suffer from ear problems may want to practice this exercise many times during the day until the condition improves.

MOUTH EXERCISES:
TONGUE, SALIVA AND TEETH CLICKING

In addition to the other areas of the face, we need to stimulate as well the mouth, gums and teeth to keep them healthy and strong. We continually use our mouths for talking, eating and kissing. The mouth exercises help keep this area strong and prevent tooth decay and gum problems such as gingivitis.

First, roll the tongue around the inside of the mouth and across the gums and teeth. We want to use the tongue as we would a toothbrush. The tongue is recognized as the opening to the heart. Feelings of hate, love, sympathy and anger reside in the heart and are stimulated by the tongue. When we kiss using the tongue, passion rises in the heart. So this exercise not only washes and cleans the mouth and teeth, but stimulates the heart as well.

As you roll the tongue around the mouth, saliva will be secreted by the salivary glands. Don't swallow it, but allow it to collect until you have a mouth full of saliva. Next, swish it around as if you were using a mouthwash. Wash the entire inside of the mouth including the gums and in between the teeth. Then divide the saliva into three equal parts and swallow each part separately and slowly until the mouth is clear. The Chinese call this the "heavenly water" and when you swallow it, feel it as it descends to the stomach. You may begin to feel the energy which it brings to the stomach.

The literal English translation of this exercise is: "The Red Dragon dances over the ocean to make the wind, rain and clouds." The Red

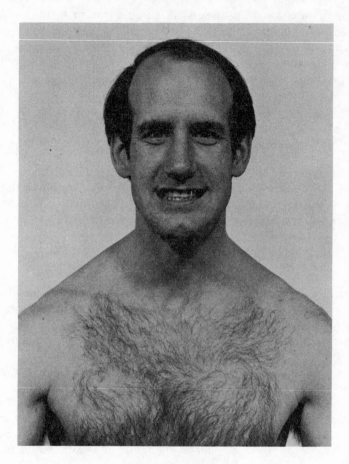

25. Teeth Click.

Dragon is the tongue and the ocean is the saliva. This saliva or heavenly water is sacred to the Taoists and is treated with respect for the power it holds as a natural healing water. Saliva helps to kill germs in the mouth and may be used as a form of medicine. It may also be used to treat infections. If you cut yourself, put the cut in your mouth or spread some of your saliva over it. The saliva will help to clean it out and destroy bacteria or germs that might otherwise lead to infection. Interestingly, it is now known that saliva triggers the production of a particular hormone within the structure of the teeth which helps to prevent tooth decay.

Further, saliva is a very important aid in digestion, and along with the teeth, forms the first step in breaking down foodstuffs before they reach the stomach. Therefore you want to stimulate your salivary glands daily to insure their continuing strength into old age. We also want to protect the teeth from decaying because if you cannot chew properly, you will not be able to digest your food properly. The resultant decreased capacity to absorb the nutritive elements from food develops into a generally weakened internal system. When you do eat, always chew your food until it is in liquid form. This insures that enough saliva penetrates the food to begin breaking it down. Remember, there are no teeth in your stomach. To exercise the teeth, we need to practice teeth clicking.

Click the teeth together thirty-six times. This strengthens the teeth and gums. When practiced in the morning, it will help awaken you, and when practiced during the day, it helps to keep you alert. A sign of old age is often loose teeth as well as loose joints. Clicking the teeth, as well as clenching the teeth during the day, will help tighten the joints of the body and keep the teeth healthy. The body tends to loosen up and become vulnerable to outside germs and bacteria during sexual intercourse, orgasm and while moving the bowels. Teeth clicking or teeth clenching during these moments helps to protect the body and keep up one's natural defenses.

There are also points at the top and bottom of the lips which may be pressed to stimulate the meridians which supply energy to the mouth, teeth and gums. Press with a firm and steady pressure and follow with a rubbing movement to energize this area. Repeat three times.

These four exercises should be practiced in the morning after performing the ear exercise, after meals, and at other appropriate times as recommended above.

RUBBING THE FACE

After all the exercises which energize the individual parts of the face have been practiced, one needs to simulate the skin and facial muscles. Begin by rubbing the palms of the hands together vigorously. Then press the palms against the face so that you feel the warmth in the hands enter into the skin and penetrate into the muscles. Use your imagination and feel the energy being absorbed by the cells throughout the face. Then rub the hands in an outward circular action around the face. Work the fingers and hands up through the bridge of the nose, through the third eye and out across the forehead, proceeding down the temples and cheeks and across

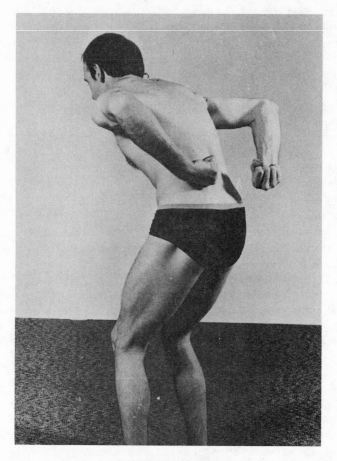

26. Kidney Exercise (1).

the chin and mouth, crossing back up along the nose. Continue to rub for as long as you feel comfortable. You may want to stop occasionally to rub the hands together to bring more heat and energy into the face. Practice this exercise whenever the facial muscles become tired. This will help to reduce the formation of wrinkles on the skin and bring a glow to your complexion.

STIMULATING THE KIDNEYS

After you have stretched the body and toes and exercised the face, sit or stand up. (This exercise may also be practiced in a prone position for those who are bedridden.) Rub the hands together vigorously to get the energy flowing to the palms and fingers. Place the palms on the small of the back. Keep the upper body tilted slightly forward. Feel as well as imagine the energy and heat flowing from the hands into the back and kidneys. Then massage the small of the back by rubbing up and down and then in a circular motion across the back. Next, clench the fingers together to form two fists and hit the small of your back with the back of your hands. Pummel the area softly for a few seconds. Then repeat the rubbing and pummeling action three times. This exercise should be done in the morning or whenever there is lower back pain.

The exercise stimulates the adrenal glands and the kidneys, which lie directly behind the small of the back. Lower back pain is often caused by a weakness in the kidneys. Two factors which help to weaken the kidneys are drinking an excess of liquids and standing on the feet for prolonged periods. By practicing this exercise you will be strengthening, energizing and healing the kidneys and the adrenals, and thus by association, you will be curing lower back problems as well as strengthening the eyes (as the kidneys are connected with the eyes). This pose also helps keep the skin smooth and beautiful and encourages strong sexual feelings by energizing the glandular system.

LIVER EXERCISE

The kidneys and the liver are the two main filters of the body. They are responsible for eliminating toxins from the blood and for maintaining the proper acid-alkaline balance within the body. So we want to practice the kidney exercise to stimulate and strengthen the adrenals and kidneys, and perform the liver exercise to keep the liver functioning properly.

Sit or lie down in a comfortable position. (Refer once again to the descriptions of the proper way to sit and stand.) Place the palm of the right hand on the right lateral side of the body so that it lies at the base of the rib cage. Push the hand across the front of the chest following the line made by the lower rib bones of the chest. Run up toward the sternum and then down toward the left lateral side of the chest. Rubbing once from the right to the left constitutes one turn. Repeat the movement 36 times. The heel of the hand should exert pressure on the skin as you rub the hand across it. The liver lies just below the skin under the rib cage on the right side of the body. The pressure exerted by the hand rubbing across the chest stimulates the flow of energy as well as the circulation of blood to the liver.

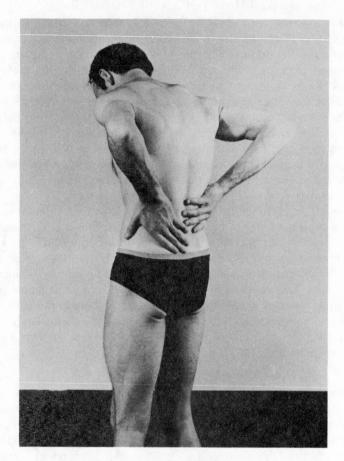

27. Kidney Exercise (2).

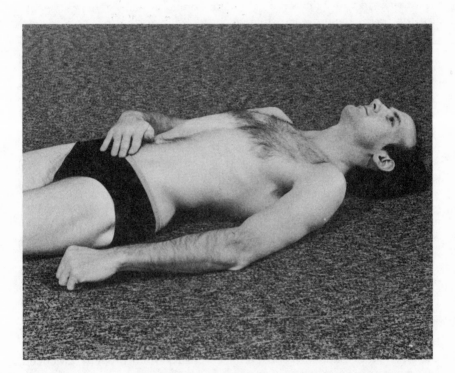

28. Solar Plexus Rubbing. (To disperse energy and to cure constipation, rub
only in a *clockwise* direction; to stimulate energy and to cure diarrhea, rub
only in a *counterclockwise* direction.)

You may also use the left hand to rub across the chest, beginning at the left lateral side and again follow the outline made by the lower ribs as you rub across the chest to the right side. The stomach lies just below the skin on the left side of the chest and so this hand rubbing keeps the energy flowing to the stomach. Do this exercise 36 times also. You may want to alternate the hands, starting first with the right hand for one turn, then using the left hand for one turn, continuing the rotation until you have performed 36 rubbings with each hand.

Practicing the two exercises helps to build up the relationship between the digestive organs, stomach and liver. You want to push the energy from one organ to the other so that the two organs will work together smoothly. Throughout this exercise, as with all the exercises, you want to keep your mind on what you are doing. It helps if you can visualize the flow of energy across your chest. Keeping the mind on the task helps to increase the benefits derived from doing the exercise as well as serving to unify the mind with the body. Practice this exercise in the morning after you have performed the kidney stimulating exercise.

Recently, while on a lecture tour, I had reason to demonstrate this exercise. I asked my audience to perform it for themselves. I noted at the time one woman who entered into the spirit of it with obvious gusto. Several weeks later, that same women telephoned my office to ask if she might fly up to see me. When she arrived — and to my great astonishment — she said she'd made the trip only to thank me. "For what," I asked. "For the liver exercise," she replied. "I have had liver trouble all my life. When you demonstrated the liver exercise at your lecture I said to myself, 'What have I got to lose?' and began doing the exercise. Two weeks later, at my regular checkup, my family physician told me my liver condition had improved sixty percent — and he couldn't imagine why. So that's why I'm here — simply to thank you!"

BRINGING FIRE INTO THE STOVE

From the original Chinese, the term "Solar Plexus Exercise" roughly translates into English as, "The fire burns the Wheel." The "Wheel" is the navel or solar plexus located in the abdominal cavity. This area contains the intestines, bladder, kidneys and adrenals. When properly practiced, this exercise creates the feeling of a fire burning in the abdominal cavity. Thus, in traditional Chinese medicine, the abdominal cavity is referred to as "the stove." Building up this fire will help to burn out every disease associated with this area of the body, including diarrhea, constipation, flatulence, diverticulitis, cancer and other disorders.

Lie on your back. Using the palm of either hand, rub in a clockwise motion starting at the navel and rubbing in increasingly larger circles. Then reverse the direction and rub in continually shrinking circles. You must continue the rubbing until the abdomen becomes hot. It is exceedingly important that you follow what you are doing in this exercise. Think about the heat building up. You will begin to feel very warm, but you need to continue the exercise until the area around your navel is burning like a fire.

If you don't feel the fire, then you haven't done it long enough. This requires a great deal of concentration and patience. Think less about your worries and more about the exercise. At first, you may find that it is seemingly impossible to practice for a long enough time to build up even a slight amount of heat. However, with practice, you will begin to feel the warmth building until you feel the energy burning from within the abdomen.

The colon runs in a transverse direction across the abdomen from the right to the left side of the body. By rubbing only in a clockwise fashion, any problems of constipation will be cured. This motion helps to disperse or push out the contents of the colon. Correspondingly, by rubbing only in a counterclockwise motion, you will tend to reabsorb excessive liquids within the colon back into the body, and this will help to cure diarrhea. If you have a healthy system, you will want to rub the abdomen in both the clockwise and counterclockwise dirctions as we have described above.

The best time to practice these exercises is in the morning when you are freshly rested and have a good supply of energy. They may be practiced again in the evening if you so desire.

RUBBING THE ARMS AND LEGS:
MERIDIAN MASSAGE

The meridians or energy channels which regulate the liver, pancreas and kidneys all come together on the inside of the thighs. These three meridians come in to energize the entire-upper channel of the body. By massaging these pathways correctly, we are able to stimulate the entire body, including the sexual organs, as these meridians pass through the pelvis on their way up the body. In a similar fashion, the gallbladder, bladder and stomach meridians run in a downward path along the outside of the leg. By massaging these pathways, we stimulate the organs and tissues associated with the meridians.

By massaging the legs on the inside in an upward manner, we stimulate the circulation of blood within the lower half of the body. People who have jobs which require them to sit or stand all day long, tend to develop cramps and varicose veins in their legs. This is because the blood tends to pool in the feet and legs, which hampers proper circulation. By stimulating the meridians of the leg, we can strengthen the healthy flow of blood and prevent future problems from developing in the legs. Likewise, by massaging the outside of the legs in a downward fashion, problems such as high blood pressure, water retention and overweight (all of which are associated with the gall-bladder, bladder and stomach meridians) can be cured or prevented from occurring. Problems of bursitis and arthritis can also be reversed or at least prevented from degenerating further.

UPWARD MASSAGE

Practice this in a standing position. (The pose may also be done while sitting or lying down.) Begin by placing the palms of the hands on

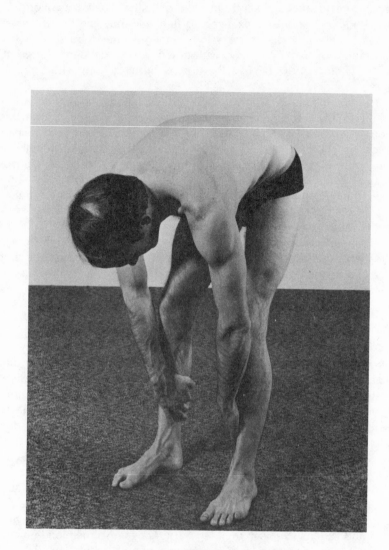

29. Leg Rubbing — upward meridians (1).

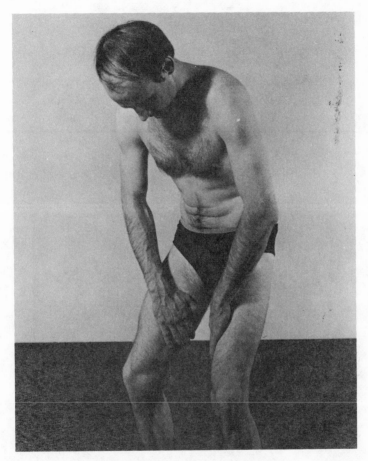

30. Leg Rubbing — upward meridians (2).

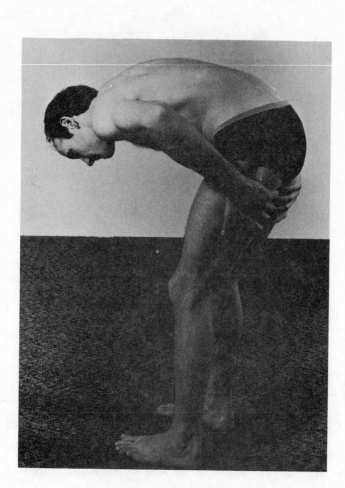

31. Leg Rubbing — downward meridians (1).

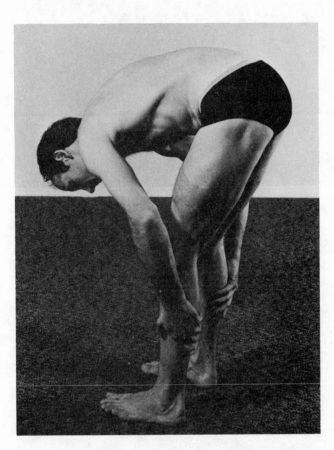

32. Leg Rubbing — downward meridians (2).

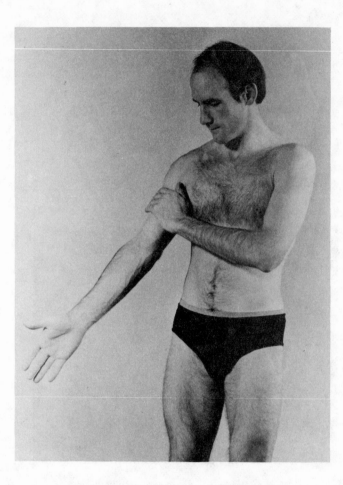

33. Arm Rubbing — downward meridians (1).

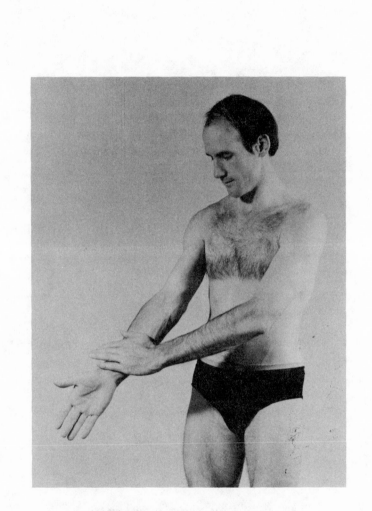

34. **Arm Rubbing — downward meridians (2).**

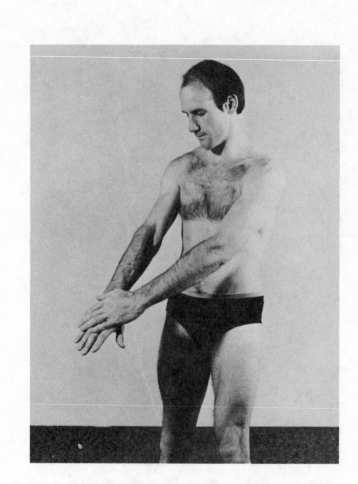

35. Arm Rubbing—upward meridians (1).

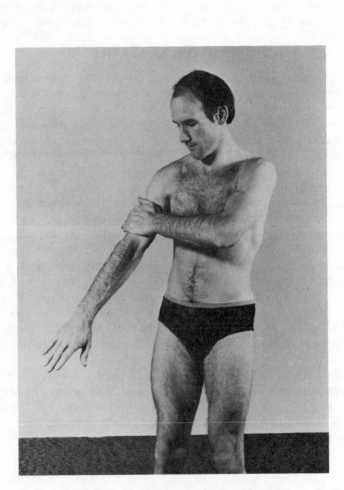

36. Arm Rubbing — upward meridians (2).

the inside of the legs at the ankles. Now slowly bring the palms up the leg, through the inside of the knees, up the thighs and into the genitals. Then begin again at the ankles and repeat the rubbing motion twelve times. At all times keep pressure on the hands so that a slight warmth may be felt as you massage the leg. Breathe normally throughout the exercise. You may also practice this exercise by just concentrating on rubbing the area from the knee to the thigh. This is the most important part of the exercise.

DOWNWARD MASSAGE

Practice this exercise in a standing position. (It may also be performed sitting or lying down if necessary.) The standing position also helps to stretch the hamstrings, knees, tendons and calves of the legs and brings energy down into the toes. Begin by placing the palms of the hands on the outside of the thighs. Now in a continuous motion, rub the hands down the legs along the outside of the knees and calves until you come to the ankles. Then repeat again for a total of twelve times. This movement helps to dispel the energy from the body — this is why it helps problems such as obesity, water retention and high blood pressure. You will not want to do this in the morning as at that time it is preferable to energize the body by practicing the upward massage only. Just breathe normally while performing this exercise.

Just as with the leg massage, you may massage the arms to stimulate the heart, lung and heart constrictor meridians which run down the inside of the arm, and the triple heater, large intestine and small intestine meridians which run up on the outside of the arms toward the shoulders. Place the left palm on the inside of the right shoulder and in a continuous motion, rub the palm down through the inside of the elbow to the tips of the fingers. Then bring the left palm over the fingers and continue to rub up the back of the hand, through the outside of the elbow onto the shoulder. Repeat this movement twelve times. Then reverse by bringing the right hand onto the left arm, and rubbing first downward on the inside of the arms, then upward along the outside of the arm. Repeat this motion twelve times also.

WEIGHT REDUCTION

Being excessively overweight is dangerous to one's health. This does not mean that it is wrong to be overweight, but merely that it goes against the natural laws of healing. Understand clearly the harm to one's health which being overweight brings, and you may lose all desire to be overweight. Blood which is normally sent to the head and brain remains in the abdominal cavity to aid the digestive organs with their increased load. The heart must work harder (and because of this excess strain, becomes critically weakened and more likely to collapse) due to the increase of fatty tissues and, usually, because of the weakened circulation in the arteries and veins as a result of fats and lipids in the blood, high blood pressure results. It is said that if your abdomen is larger than your chest, you can buy a box to prepare for your funeral. Excessive weight brings on physical

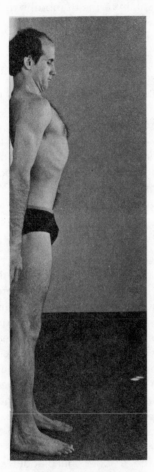

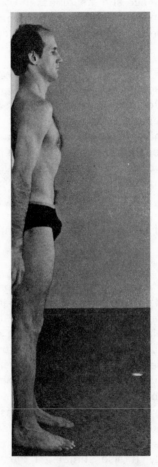

37. Weight Reducing (1). **38. Weight Reducing (2).**

as well as mental fatigue and sluggishness caused by the system being constantly overworked. There is usually accompanying lower back pain due to the increased load on the spine. The weight reduction exercise helps to bring down the weight to a manageable level and helps adjust the back to keep it healthy and strong. When practicing this exercise, remember never to force yourself or push beyond your limitations. Acquire patience and steadiness in your practice. Think in terms of months rather than days and you will be able to bring down your excessive weight and tone the body to a normal level of health.

Part One

First, stand against a wall so the heels, buttocks, upper back and head lie against the wall. Inhaling through the nose, stretch the body upward and pull the abdomen in as far as possible so the chest expands fully. Keep the arms by your sides. The shoulders should feel as if they are expanding and pressing against the wall. Now exhale as quickly as possible through the mouth. Blow the breath out fully and push the abdomen outward. The entire body will tighten automatically on the exhale if done properly. Practice this inhale-exhale repetition seven to twelve times. You will find that with consistent practice, the muscles in the abdomen and body will tighten and become toned and strengthened. Excess fat, water and flesh muscle will be eliminated, and the belly will shrink.

Part Two

Stand away from the wall and bring the heels off the floor so that you will be standing as high on the toes as possible. Keep the spine erect and straight, and bend the knees slightly as if you were to bring the thighs parallel to the floor and sink slowly down as if you were going to sit on a chair. The arms will fall at a 45° angle from the body. Keep the breath regular, and stay in the pose from ten to twenty seconds, or longer if possible. At first it will be impossible to keep the back straight and the heels up very far. With patience and practice, you will be able to get the heels perpendicular to the floor, the thighs parallel to the floor, and the back straight. This pose strengthens and tones the thighs, calves and ankles. It makes the abdominal muscles strong and increases the circulation in the legs and body, as well as strengthening the back and the nerves in the body. It also stimulates the meridians of the bladder, gallbladder and stomach. These meridians lie along the legs, and so it helps to reduce water retention and excessive weight and lowers the blood pressure. Always practice both parts of the exercise at the same sitting as they balance and compliment each other.

THE LOWER BACK

Pain itself is not a disease but is rather a signal of an existing or developing problem. Lower back pain is no exception. Lumbago, lordosos, slipped discs and other back problems limit movement and create unnecessary pain. The Lower Back exercise is designed to strengthen the spine, the muscles around the abdomen, vertebrae, tail bones and the kidneys. When done daily, it helps to cure lower back problems.

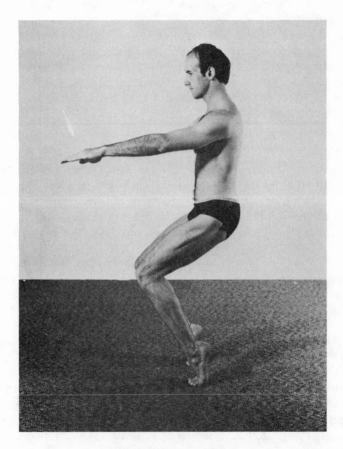

39. Weight Reducing (3).

Assume a sitting position and bring the knees up into the chest. Hold around the knees with the hands. If possible, grab onto the elbows with each hand. As you inhale, straighten the spine and lift the head upward. Then as you exhale, hunch the back so the lower abdomen becomes like a ball — as if you were about to roll over backward. The head will come forward toward the knees. Repeat this straightening and hunching movement seven times. Seven is the number of creation and this exercise will help to create a new back. Practice all the movements slowly, with your full concentration on your lower back.

This exercise may also be done while lying on your back. Place one hand under your lower back and feel the hollow space under the lower spine. Tuck under the tail bone and drop the lower back to the floor as much as possible. When you have pressed the back to the floor, release your back to the beginning position, and start again. Repeat this process seven times for one cycle.

HEALING THE STOMACH

Sit in a comfortable position, preferably on a chair with the feet flat on the floor, the thighs parallel to the floor and the spine erect and straight. Place the left palm on the stomach. As you inhale, slowly move the palm of the right hand away from the chest. One's concentration should focus upon the heel of the hand. As you push the hand and the arm forward, imagine that you are pushing away a heavy object with the heel of the hand. The eyes should follow the movements of the right hand intently throughout this exercise. Then, as you exhale, slowly bring the right hand back into the chest. Perform this in-and-out movement seven times each time you do this exercise.

This exercise helps to cure stomach pain, ulcers, over-acidity, flatulence and stomach cancer. It helps to take the attention of the mind away from the stomach. As you move the hand away from the chest, hold in your attention or actually visualize the bad energy of the body moving out of the stomach. A circle of energy is created as new energy comes into the stomach through the left hand and diseased energy comes out through the right hand. To be effective, this exercise requires a deep meditation on what you are doing. It should be practiced slowly, with total synchronization of the breath, mind and movement of the hands.

HEART EXERCISE

Lie down on a firm surface so only the left lateral side of your body is touching the surface. (This exercise may only be practiced lying on the left side.) Extend the left arm so that it lies straight along the left side of the body with the hand down toward the left knee. The left arm will press firmly into the chest and heart region as the body lies on top of it. The left leg should be straight with the right knee bent slightly. The right arm will lie gently down on the floor in front of the body with the hand a little bit above the head. Allow the head and face to relax on the floor. The left arm should exert quite a bit of pressure on the heart so that during the exer-

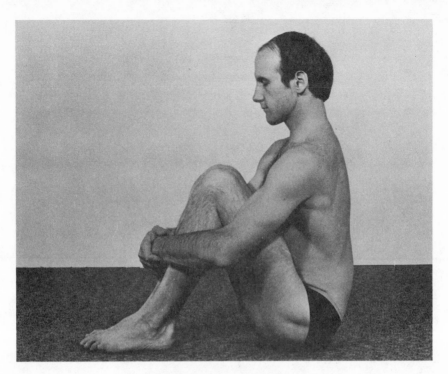

40. Lower Back Exercise (1).

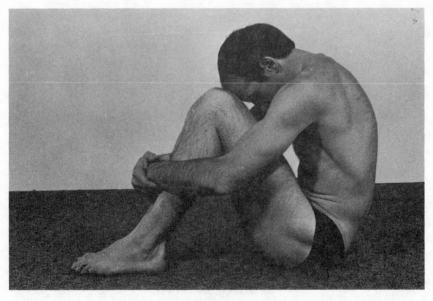

41. Lower Back Exercise (2).

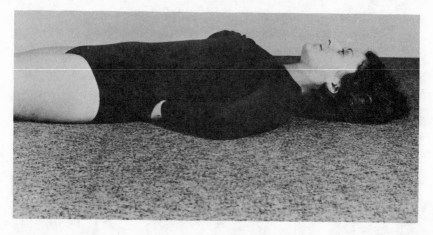

42. Lower Back Exercise (3).

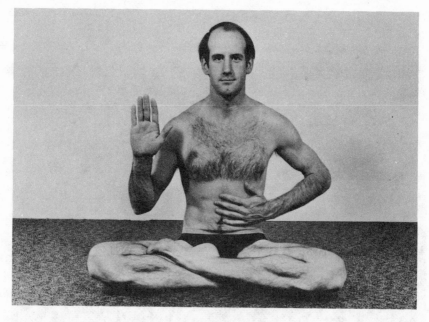

43. Healing Stomach (1).

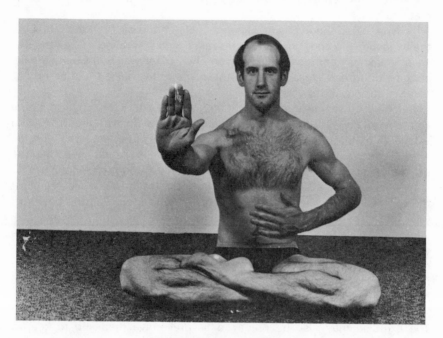

44. Healing Stomach (2).

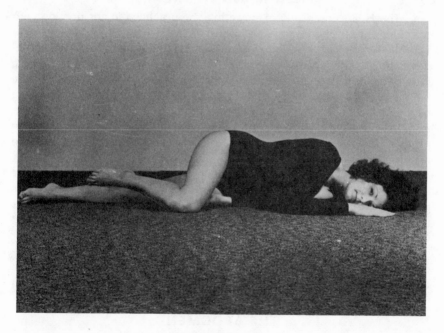

45. Heart Exercise.

cise the heart remains constricted. This prevents the heart from over-reacting.

Now close the eyes and slowly exhale all the air from the lungs. As the air leaves the body, imagine or visualize with your mind that all the disease, weakness and pain is leaving the heart. Then as you slowly inhale, imagine that fresh, clean energy is entering into the heart and that it is becoming strong and revitalized.

You may visualize, as you inhale, that a white mist or warm steam comes into the heart, penetrating every crevice within the heart. As you exhale, think that the weakness and disease goes out of the heart with the steam. You want to wash out the heart. At all times the inhalation and the exhalation should be very slow and done only through the nose.

This exercise cures diseases and problems of the heart. However, for the exercise to be effective, you must concentrate with all the power of your mind. If you find that your mind has wandered during the exercise, begin again. Perform the inhale-exhale repetition seven times each time you practice this exercise. The Heart exercise may be practiced morning, noon and night, depending upon the seriousness of the problem. If you have a weak heart, practice it once a day. If there are palpitations of the heart or angina, practice it at least twice a day. If you have had a heart attack, then this exercise needs to be performed at least three times a day. The exercise may also be practiced as preventive medicine to keep a strong heart healthy.

ENERGIZING THE HEART

The Heart Energizing exercise may be practiced in conjunction with or separate from the Heart exercise. Sit or stand in a comfortable position with the hands extended out in front of the chest at the level of the shoulders. The finger tips of each hand should almost come together, but keep a little distance between them. Keep the eyes foucused on the tips of the fingers or close them gently. See if you can feel a current of energy flowing between the fingers, from one hand to the other. Hold the arms out in front of you as long as you comfortably can, and keep your concentration on the energy flow. Let the arms relax for a few minutes, then repeat the exercise a total of three times.

This exercise creates a flow of energy which comes in through the fingers of the right hand, comes across the chest and into the heart, then passes out through the left arm, hand and fingers. As the energy passes through the heart, it strengthens the heart tissue and surrounding blood vessels. If at first you are unable to perceive the energy flow, develop your patience and keep practicing the exercise. You will quickly begin to perceive a tinglIng sensation in the finger tips. With practice, you will be able to feel the entire circle of energy as it passes through the arms, body and heart. Then you will know that you are building a strong heart.

THE ABDOMEN

Begin this exercise in a standing position, with the arms stretched out in front of the body and held slightly above the chest. Inhale completely, so that the lungs fill with air and the chest expands. Now begin to

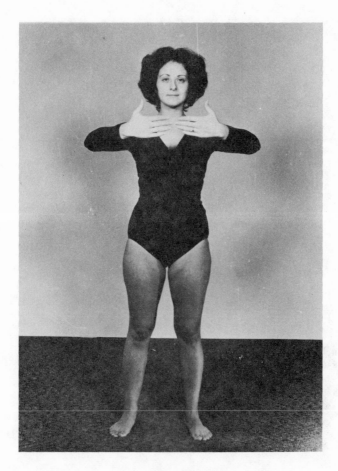

46. Energizing the Heart.

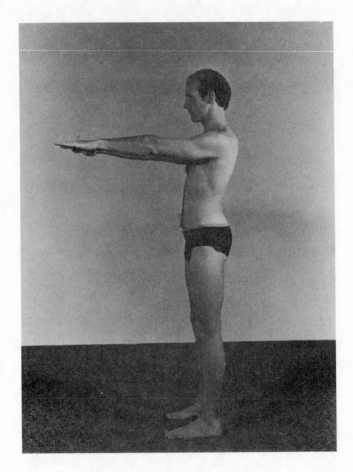

47. Abdominal Strengthening (1).

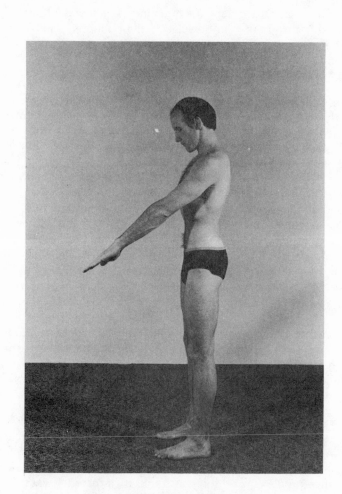

48. Abdominal Strengthening (2).

exhale slowly, using only the abdominal muscles to force the air out of the lungs. As you exhale, slowly drop the arms down to your side and tighten the abdominal muscles as much as possible. As you begin your next inhalation, bring the arms in front of you again. Repeat the exercise seven times.

This exercise strengthens the intestines, colon and internal organs in the abdomen. It tightens the muscles of the abdomen and helps to cure such problems as constipation and diarrhea. It also adjusts the posture and strengthens the spine.

THE LUNGS

Begin in a standing position with the back straight, chin slightly into the chest, head erect (as if the back of the neck is stretching upward) with the feet shoulder-width apart and parallel to each other. Now exhale all the air from the lungs and clasp the hands behind your back. Inhale slowly, expanding the lungs and pushing your hands (which are behind you) away from your back. Keep the chin tucked into the chest and use only the chest to breathe with while practicing this exercise. As you exhale, drop the hands and bring the arms out in front of you. Continue to raise the arms, bringing the hands up toward the head and then around behind the back and back up in front of the body to form one cycle. The fingers should be pointed throughout the rotation. Then interlace the fingers behind the back and begin the exercise again on the inhalation. Do this exercise seven times.

As you inhale the air into the lungs, think about fresh energy coming in to invigorate the lung tissues. As you exhale, imagine that all the germs, stale air and toxins are leaving the lungs. This exercise helps to heal any kind of lung problem, even a common cold. It strengthens the entire breathing system, including the skin (which is often referred to as the "third lung").

SEXUAL GLANDS AND LOWER BODY

Primary symptoms of old age are often experienced as coldness or numbness in the legs and feet due to the deterioration of the circulatory system at the extremities of the body, stiffness of the joints, and the lack of sexual energy. This exercise is designed to reverse these and other degenerative problems of the lower trunk, thus restoring youthfulness to the body. The pose increases the circulation to the toes, feet and legs as well as all the organs throughout the abdomen. It frees up the pelvis and joints of the knees and ankles, strengthens the nerves throughout the lower trunk of the body and stimulates the kidney, liver and spleen-pancreas meridians which pass up on the inside of the legs and into the sexual glands. It works to cure sexual problems such as impotence, premature ejaculation and other problems of retardation, as well as menstrual problems of the female system such as cramps and excessive bleeding. It is also an excellent exercise for pregnant women as it opens up the pelvis and assures an easy delivery.

Sit on the floor and bend the knees so that the soles of the feet come together in front of your body. First rub the bottoms of the feet together

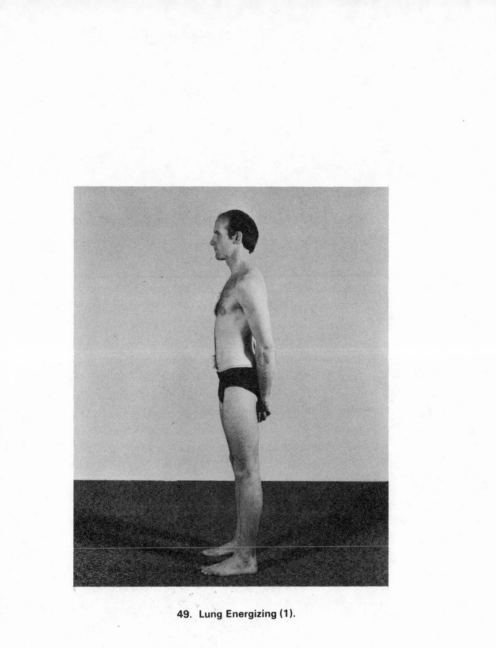

49. Lung Energizing (1).

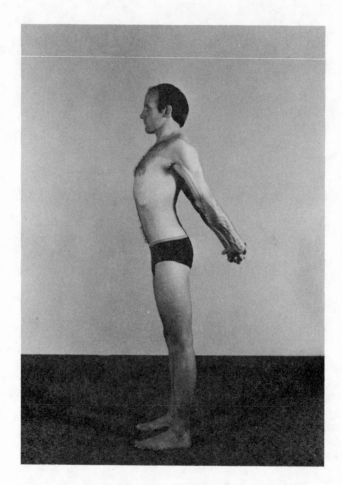

50. Lung Energizing (2).

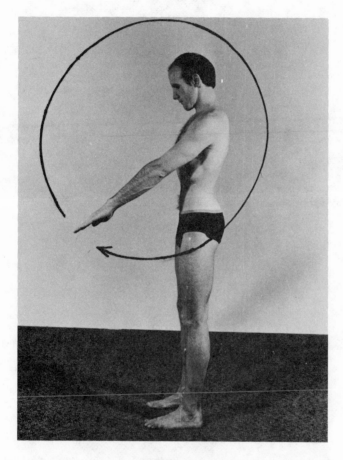

51. Lung Energizing (3).

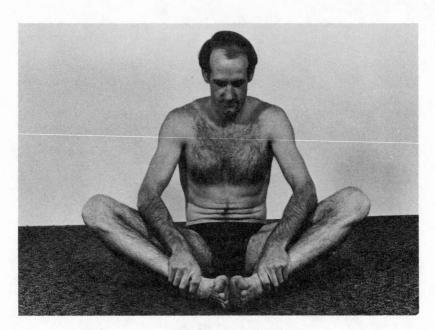

52. Six Glands Exercise (1).

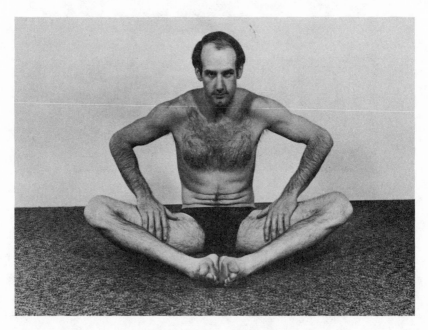

53. Six Glands Exercise (2).

until they are warm and then touch them together. Next, rub the toes with the fingers to stimulate the circulation in the feet. Then, with the feet together, draw the heels as close into the pelvis as you can get them. Begin to work the knees down toward the floor by pressing the elbows in against the thighs while holding onto the toes with the hands. Do not force the knees down; just allow the muscles to relax as you push them down. Then, using the palms of the hands, rub the inside of the thighs starting at the knees, massaging upward to the inner pelvis. This will stimulate the liver, kidney and spleen-pancreas meridians. Repeat this massaging action seven times. After this is done, gently beat on the inner thighs with the fists. This will stimulate the circulation of blood and energy in the legs and sexual organs. Continue to work with the exercise as long as you feel comfortable.

PAIN RELIEF

This simple exercise helps to relieve upper back, shoulder or neck pain and may be practiced whenever discomfort is felt in the upper spine.

Assume the proper position for sitting. If pain is felt in the upper right quadrant of the back, allow the right arm to lie motionless on the thighs. (You should of course reverse the arms if the pain is on the left side.) Extend the left arm out in front of the chest with the fingers pointed. Fix the eyes on the fingers of the left hand and slowly begin to move the left hand up and out to your left side. Keep the breathing normal, and raise the arm as high as possible. Then slowly lower the left arm to its original position and repeat the movement seven times. The exercise helps to remove the attention away from the pain in the upper trunk and brings healing energy into the sore area. Throughout the exercise, keep your attention focused on the hand that is being raised. If your mind wanders, then bring it back to your hand. You may wish to synchronize the breathing with the hand raising, in which case inhale as the arm moves upward, and exhale as you bring the arm down.

THE HANDS, ARMS AND UPPER BODY
Part One

This exercise is similar to ones practiced in T'ai Chi, Kung Fu and Karate. The pose builds up the strength of the arms and hands, tones the muscles and nerves of the arms, increases the circulation of the blood and energizes the heart, lungs and heart constrictor meridians which lie along the arm. The secret of this exercise is that it increases the energy within the arm, not just the bulk of the muscles. By concentrating on the flow of energy within the arms and hands, your arms will grow strong and will therefore tire less when you are performing manual tasks. This exercise helps to heal all problems of the arms, including arthritis, bursitis and tennis elbow.

This exercise may be practiced sitting, standing or lying down. Begin with the right hand in close to the right armpit with the palm facing frontward. Slowly move the hand away from the chest and extend it straight out, leading with the heel of the hand. Keep the fingers relaxed, and

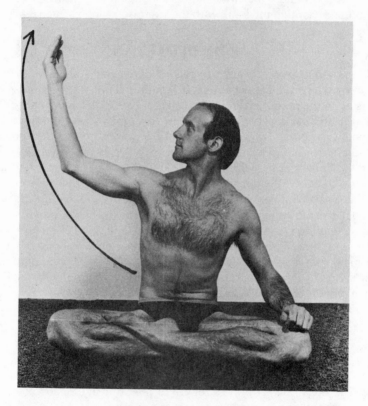

54. Pain Relief Exercise.

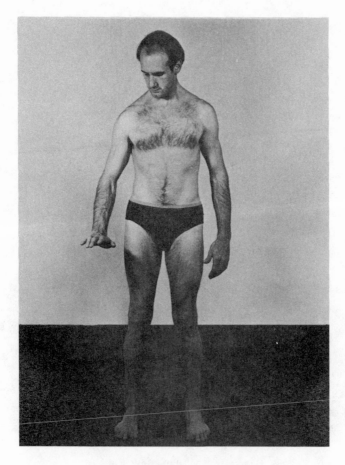

55. Hand and Arm Exercise.

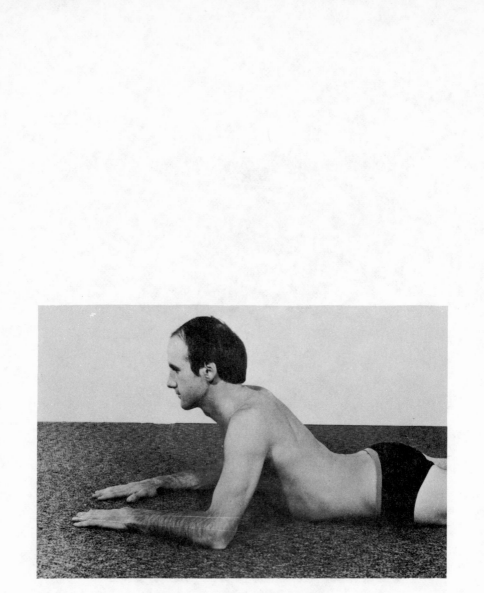

56. Hand, Arm and Upper Body Exercise.

breathing normally, try to feel that you are pushing the air away from the body. Repeat this movement seven times, and then perform the exercise with the left hand.

When practicing the arm and hand pressing exercise, never force the movements. Use little pressure and feel that the hands are like velvet, warm and full of energy, and firm but soft. Always concentrate fully on what you are doing, otherwise you will not be able to stimulate the energy so that it flows properly through the arm, wrist and hand.

Part Two

This exercise, like the one before it, is used to energize and strengthen the arms and hands. These are subtle but very dynamic exercises which may be easily overlooked, but which, when practiced, bring many beneficial results. The Arm exercise also helps to heal problems associated with the shoulder, arms and hands and works to kill the pain accompanying such problems as tennis elbow, bursitis and arthritis. Practice this exercise when you have pain in any part of the upper limbs and continue the treatment until you have regained the complete mobility of the injured part.

Lie down on the floor on your stomach and place your palms on the floor shoulder-width apart and slightly in front of each shoulder. The forearms and elbows should remain on the floor throughout the exercise. Keep the chest and head up off the floor and your breathing normal. Allow the legs to relax and keep a light but steady pressure on the arms. Now imagine that you are walking with your arms much like a soldier would do while crawling across a field on his stomach. Actually, you will not move your arms at all — simply use your imagination. Hold this position for several seconds with a deep and concentrated attention. Then relax your mind and turn the head back to look at the heel of the right foot. As you inhale, imagine that the air comes in through that foot, travels up the leg and through your body so that it comes into your right arm and down to your fingers. Then as you exhale, send the air back out the arm and down the right leg so that it leaves the body through the right foot. Then turn the head the other way and repeat the breathing using the left foot, leg and arm to follow the air through the body. Repeat the total exercise seven times each time you practice it.

Through the use of the breathing and deep concentration, you will be stimulating the energy meridians along the legs and arms which supply energy to the upper limbs. By practicing this exercise, you will not only be increasing the flow of energy to the upper body, but you will also be increasing the circulation of blood as well. For the exercise to be effective, you must concentrate deeply for the duration of the exercise. If you find that your mind wanders during the process, then begin again. At first you will not be able to detect the flow of energy through the body, but with practice, you will come to feel the energy as it enters the foot, travels up the leg and enters into the arm and hands. The inflow of energy will help to heal any injury or disease you may have in your arms or shoulders.

4 *Taoist Meditations and Breathing*

In addition to the physical and cultural exercises, the ancient Taoists discovered invaluable methods of meditation and breathing such as the Meridian Meditation and Brain Cleansing Breathing exercises, which they used to augment the energy within their bodies, to help provide for a constant and unimpeded flow of energy along the meridians, as well as providing a tool for observing inner states of weakness and disease. They also discovered practical contemplative exercises such as the Sunlight and North Star Contemplations, which were used to focus their energy in desired directions toward specific goals such as a new job or financial security or to cultivate peace of mind.

The Taoists also developed meditations and breathing techniques which are concerned with transmuting the flow of the generative energy. Instead of being discharged to procreate offspring or to waste away, it is retained in the body for purification and transmutation into positive vitality, thus restoring within us the original spirit which existed before we came into being and which exists all around and within us presently. These techniques, called Immortal Breathing and the Small and Large Heavenly Cycles, are a series of comprehensive methods designed to create an alchemical change within the practitioner to bring him or her into a final state of self-realization and immortality.

We have included four of these basic techniques in this chapter. The serious student is directed to Lu K'Uan Lu's book, *Taoist Yoga: Alchemy and Immortality* for further studies in Immortal Breathing. The reader may also feel free to contact us through our publisher for further information.

The Taoist exercises, including the physical, meditative, contemplative and Immortal Breathing techniques, are aimed at the unification of the mind and the body with the subsequent unfolding of man into his natural state of enlightenment and immortality. The first step in all the Internal Exercises encourages the practitioner to do something, to take some kind of action either through specific physical, visual or concentrative tasks. However, the aim of the ancient Taoists was to enable each man to go beyond action into the Tao, or a state of non-attachment to action. The practice of the breathing and meditative aspects of the Internal Exercises leads one into a realization of this second step — that of non-action.

Realizing the Tao is thought to occur in three stages. The first stage is the state of individual action called eu-wei (無為). By understanding that in every action there is non-action and that in every state of non-action there is action, we come to the second state of understanding which in Chinese is called wu-wei (無不為), literally meaning, no action — acting, but with no action. However, for the entering into the Tao to occur, one must transcend the individual self, the ego or I, and enter into the third state of natural action called wu-bu-wei (有為), where action and non-action occur simultaneously in a state beyond the ego. In this state one transcends even the Tao as we know it, or think we know it — the description we have of the world, or the way we think about anything, is never the actual event in its totality.

> The Tao that can be told is not the eternal Tao.
> The name that can be named is not the eternal name.
> The nameless is the beginning of heaven and earth.
> The named is the mother of ten thousand things.
> Ever desireless, one can see the mystery.
> Ever desiring, one can see the manifestations.
> These two spring from the same source but differ in
>   name; this appears as darkness.
> Darkness within darkness.
> The gate to all mystery
>
> Tao Te Ching I

These three stages are in fact inseparable. They may be thought of as the three parts of a coin, the two sides and the middle. By practicing the Internal Exercises, man prepares himself for this final transformation which occurs in a state beyond time and space, in which every man realizes his true natural place in the universe.

> In the pursuit of learning, every day something is acquired.
> In the pursuit of the Tao, every day something is dropped.
> Less and less is done
> Until non-action is achieved.
> When nothing is done, nothing is left undone.
> The world is ruled by letting things take their course.
> It cannot be ruled by interfering.
>
> Tao Te Ching XLVIII

MERIDIAN MEDITATION

Utilizing the pathways of energy which already exist in the body, Meridian Meditation enables its practitioner to turn her/his eyes inward to her/his own body and detect states of weakness as if she/he were seeing them clearly with her/his eyes. Once properly versed in this discipline, no one will be better equipped than you to diagnose your own state of physical health.

Modern day machines and analytical techniques (X-ray, scanners, blood analysis and urine analysis, etc.) are useful in diagnosing certain diseases, but they are unable to detect many ailments such as nerve and energy problems which subtly weaken organs and tissues and later lead to complex medical problems. Weakness *is* the first step toward disease. If we have no weaknesses, then it will be impossible to contract a serious illness. Through the technique of Meridian Meditation we are able to enter into our own energy pathways and become one with ourselves. Then when we discover a problem such as an energy blockage, we can use the different modes of healing available to us such as Internal Exercises, herbs, acupuncture, meditation, and when necessary, surgery.

Meridian Meditation can often be used to uncover the origins of a weakness first thought to be located in another point in the body. A case in point is illustrated by the time I was plagued with a harsh and constant cough which was irritating the mucous linings in my throat, thus making it exceedingly difficult for me to talk. At first I thought this was due to a problem within the lungs and took appropriate herbs to treat what I thought to be the source of my problem. When the irritation still did not disperse, I suspected something else might be wrong. Using the Meridian Meditation, I observed that the origin of the problem was not in my lungs, but in my heart, the organ which supports the lungs. And so, after using a different set of herbs to treat the heart, the cough began to abate the next day. The Meridian Meditation can also be practiced as a preventive technique. It gives the student a method to discern states of weakness before they become major diseases. For example, cancer takes many years to manifest into its outward form. The inner observation one gains through Meridian Meditation can help to prevent it at its onset. Thus, this method of self-diagnosis helps a person to see all the signs before a disease begins to take hold in the body.

Meridian Meditation is also a system of self-healing. By meditating on sites within the body where energy has become blocked, it is possible to reestablish an unimpeded flow of energy at this point. We can learn to help heal others as well. Our body is a microcosm of the universe. By understanding and becoming totally familiar with this limited system, we are then capable of knowing the universal macrocosm outside ourselves. Once we are capable of traveling freely through the network of energy within our own body, we will be able to travel in the network of energy outside our body as well and thus, if we wish, to where another person is even if they are far away. *Energy is not limited by space or time.* By understanding our own patterns of energy movement, we can send out our energy in an emergency to help heal another.

Meridian Meditation has been used as a method for both physical and spiritual development for thousands of years. The venerated sage and philosopher, Lao-Tzu, purportedly lived anywhere from 160 to 500 years. He faithfully practiced, and strongly advocated the practice of Meridian Meditation to his disciples. Its mastery may take from six months to ten years, but it is worth the dedication of time and devotion to learn this method of inner observation.

Meridian Meditation is learned in three stages: 1. The Around-the-World Massage, 2. Using one's imagination, and 3. Feeling the energy flowing.

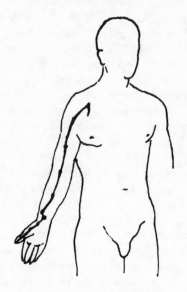

Fig. 11.   Lung Meridian.

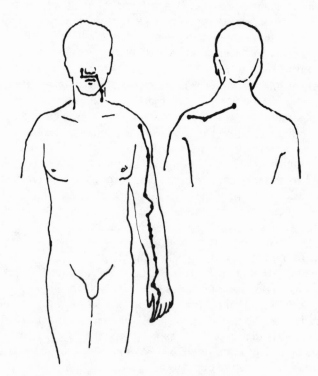

Fig. 12.   Large Intestine Meridian.

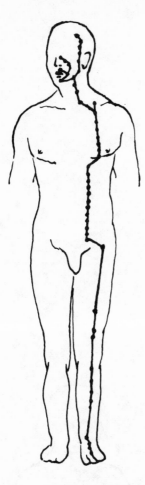

Fig. 13.   Stomach Meridian.

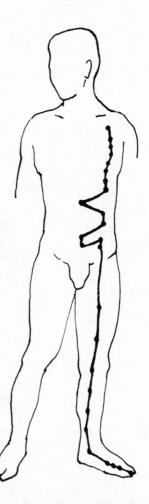

Fig. 14.   Spleen-Pancreas Meridian.

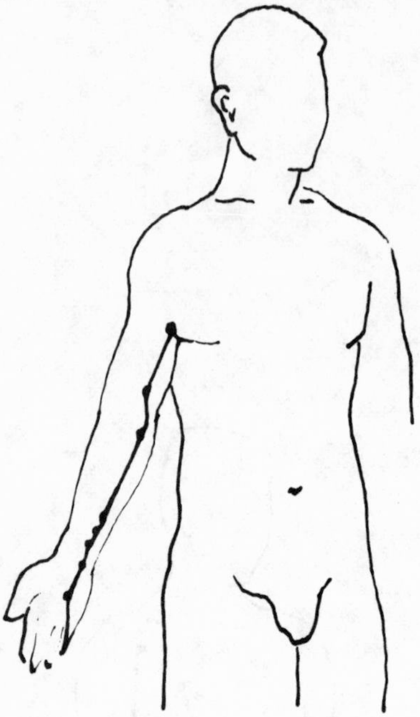

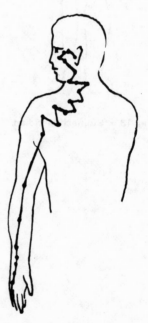

Fig. 15.   Heart Meridian.

Fig. 16.   Small Intestine Meridian.

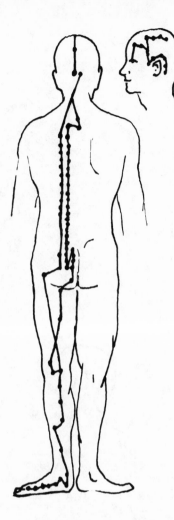

Fig. 17.   Bladder Meridian.

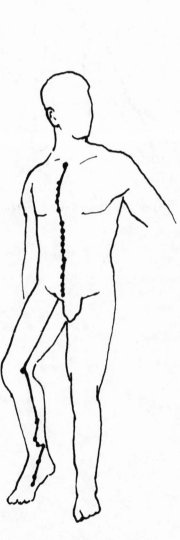

Fig. 18.   Kidney Meidian.

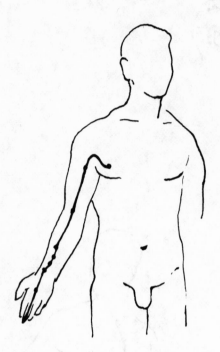

Fig. 19.   Heart Constrictor Meridian.

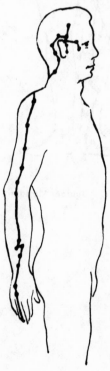

Fig. 20.   Triple Heater Meridian.

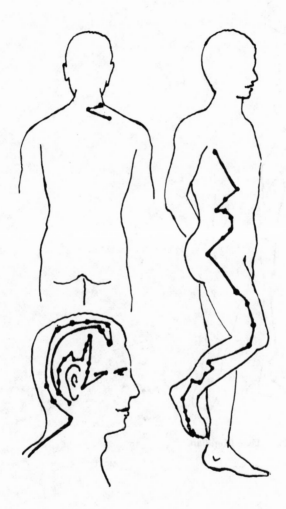

Fig. 21.   Gall Bladder Meridian.

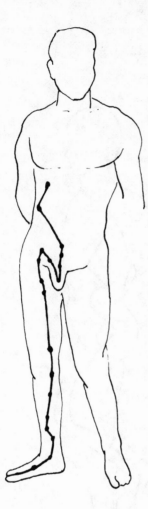

Fig. 22.   Liver Meridian.

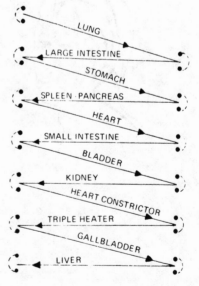

LUNG

LARGE INTESTINE

STOMACH

SPLEEN-PANCREAS

HEART

SMALL INTESTINE

BLADDER

KIDNEY

HEART CONSTRICTOR

TRIPLE HEATER

GALLBLADDER

LIVER

Fig. 23.   Sequence of Energy Flow.

The Around-the-World Massage stimulates the energy along all of the major meridians, thereby concurrently affecting the energy in all areas adjacent to those meridians. Applying this technique will enable you to become acquainted simultaneously with both paths of the main meridians — an absolute necessity for aspiring practitioners — and to intimately experience the exhilarating effects of this simple method of massage.

Using the bulb of the thumb or the tips of the index and middle fingers, gently massage the entire length of the main meridians, *in the direction of the flow of energy.* It is advised that the meridians be massaged in the prescribed sequence as they are illustrated in the figures and not in any haphazard, random order. The reason for this should be ovious; the purpose of the Meridian Massage is to stimulate and create an unbroken circle of energy circulating within the body, and this can only be accomplished by massaging the meridians in the prescribed sequence. Baby oil, massage lotions, ginger juice, etc., may be used to lubricate the surface of the skin, although this is not necessary for successfully applying the technique.

After becoming thoroughly acquainted with the paths of the twelve main meridians and with the flow of energy within the body as a result of the preceeding meridian massage, one may commence to use the imagination to trace the energy through the meridians. The correct method is to first find a comfortable position, either lying or sitting down. Sitting on a soft cushion is preferable; keep the spinal column straight so that the tail bone and the spinal column at the waist are in line. One's shoulders and back should be relaxed, however, so that the shoulders automatically fall into their natural position, which is slightly forward. This allows for maximum expansion of the lungs. Place the hands on the legs with the thumbs folded inside the palms. Empty the mind of all irrelevant, excess thoughts and focus all of your attention upon the lung meridian. You may want to begin by tracing the path of the lung meridian with your fingers, as in the Meridian Massage, paying close attention to the subjective feeling that arises as a result of this procedure. Then keep your hands on your legs and use your imagination to follow the meridian lines as you have learned them. Imagine that you feel a flow of energy descending down your arm along the lung meridian. Continue to repeat this procedure along the large intestine meridian and subsequent meridians in their appropriate order. After a number of practice sessions, you will begin to perceive the flow of energy along the meridians.

These first two techniques will eventually allow the practitioner to sense even the most minute energy fluctuations along the meridian circuit. Ultimately one will be able to willfully direct the energy flow along any one of the meridians. Becoming consciously aware of the circulation of energy within the body will enable one to maintain a state of energy balance under any and all circumstances. Disease can only inhabit a body in which there is an erratic flow of energy along the meridians.

Occasionally, as you begin your practice, you will sense an energy blockage where it will be difficult to follow the energy along the particular meridian you are tracing. For example, you may feel the energy flowing down the arm on the lung meridian, but it may stop when you get to the elbow. Thus you will know that you have a blockage of some sort. Begin again at the upper arm and retrace the flow. If it blocks again, begin again until you feel an unimpeded flow of energy. This may take several attempts or it may take weeks to get past this area. However, when you do feel that the energy is flowing smoothly and freely, you will know that you have effectively prevented or cured a weakness or disease within yourself. If the energy does not flow properly after a number of attempts at one sitting, go on to trace out the flow of energy throughout the other meridians. Then, either when you have finished or at another sitting you may return to the energy block.

Always keep in mind what you are doing. If the mind wanders, then start again from the beginning. Don't be anxious to hurry the process. First think where the energy is going and don't interrupt your thinking process. Eventually you will be able to very directly feel the flow of energy. But we need to learn to make our way around the inner world before we can learn to make our way around the universe. By practicing this method of meditation, you will learn how to unify the mind and the body in your personal microcosm. Then it will be possible to "know" the universal macrocosm that lies beyond your apparent physical limitations. The mind, the microcosm and the macrocosm will become unified, thus making clear the saying, "I am that I am."

CONTEMPLATIVE EXERCISES FOR PRACTICAL PURPOSES

A person may practice the North Star meditation, Candlelight, Moonlight or Sunlight contemplations for practical as well as for healing purposes. One may be in need of a job, money, intelligence or love. For example, if one wanted to find a new job, she would imagine that the light entering into her head *is* the new job. She would put all her wishes and hopes into the meditation. It is not necessary to even know specifically what the new job is to be. If you are correctly able to perform the meditation and experience the golden light throughout your body, then you will already have the new job, even though you don't have it yet!

In a similar manner one may fill himself up with money, intelligence, happiness, love or any other need that one may have. This is a very practical and useful exercise. As with all of the Internal Exercises, and the breathing and meditation techniques, one must experience them to understand and appreciate their simple but profound effects. The ancient Taoists were very practical people. If something worked well, they used it. If it did not, they discarded it. And this system of Internal Exercise has been around for over 6,000 years!

SUNLIGHT CONTEMPLATION

Sunlight represents a positive, energizing force which we can harness to help cleanse our bodies as well as our minds. Sunlight enables the skin of our bodies to produce Vitamin D, a necessary nutrient for good health. The combination of fresh air and sunlight has been used throughout the ages as a tonic for many ailments of the body. The Sunlight Con-

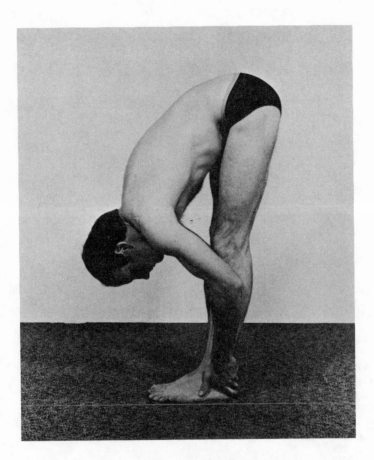

57. Sunlight Contemplation (1).

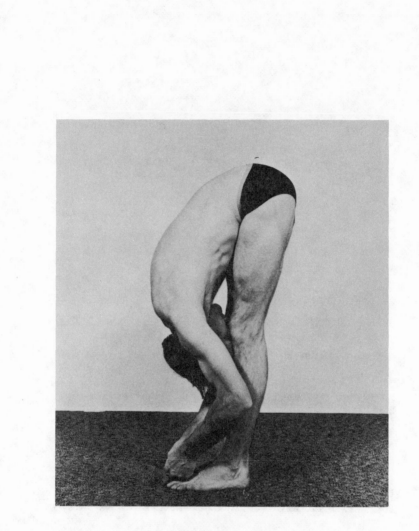

58. Sunlight Contemplation (2).

templation exercise combines the benefits of the proper breathing and visualization techniques with the health-enhancing qualities of the sun into one exercise. It works to wash the body both on the outside and on the inside, cleaning out disease and germs and restoring a feeling of vibrant and glowing health. Normally we clean our mouth and teeth as well as the rest of the body when we wash, but we never really think to clean the rectum and anus thoroughly. This negligence can cause an accumulation of germs at the anal opening, causing weakness to occur and possibly hemorrhoids, polypi or cancer of the colon or anus. Sunlight is an ever present and free source of energy which we can bathe ourselves in to wash out all disease and weaknesses and restore our energy to its proper level.

Turn the body so the spine faces the sun and lean over so that the sunlight is allowed to come into the anal opening. (This exercise needs to be done nude for the best results.) Practice the anal squeezing exercise and as you exhale, imagine that all the germs, disease and weaknesses of the body are leaving through the anal opening. Then as you inhale, imagine that the sunlight and all the energy from the sun comes in to fill up the abdomen, spine, head and entire body. Feel the warmth of the sunlight on your body and imagine that it is sterilizing the body and making it healthy, clean and fresh. Use your breathing and imagination as a contemplative exercise. Practice the entire sequence a total of seven times, performing each movement very slowly and gently. You may also practice this exercise lying down, but make sure that the sexual organs and anal opening are bathed in the sunlight.

It is not necessary to do this exercise out-of-doors. When I [Rick Miller] lived in San Francisco, the street was so narrow that my apartment looked onto a house across the street. Each morning, I could observe my Chinese neighbor on his bed. The morning sun would come through his window and he would lie for up to an hour with his back to the sun. I observed this ritual for five years before learning this Sunlight Contemplation and realizing what that gentleman had been doing every morning for all those years!

THE NORTH STAR CONTEMPLATION

The North Star is the guide star of the heavens and has been used for centuries by travelers to pinpoint their location and insure that their routes of travel were correct. It has been symbolized as the King, the Emperor or the highest place, and has been given the special name "Purple Rose" because of its beautiful purple aura. It is fitting that the Chinese have used it for thousands of years in a contemplative exercise they use for healing purposes.

Begin by sitting facing the North Star, which may be located by first finding the Big Dipper. Use your imagination and feel that the light of the North Star comes down and meets you on the top of your head at a place called "the meeting of all points." This point lies at the crown of the head at a point equidistant between the ears. Imagine that the energy from the "Purple Rose" meets your energy at this point and that this area of your head turns into a golden fire. The meridians of your body will begin to feel transparent and golden. Imagine that all the golden light penetrates throughout your entire body and down to the toes.

It is often extremely difficult to practice this exercise, as you need complete attention on what you are doing for it to be successful. If your attention wanders or you are interrupted, start again. However, never force yourself to perform the meditation. If you are unable to complete it successfully, stop and come back to it another time. Eventually you will meet with success. Once you are able to complete the meditation and feel the golden light entering your body, you may discover that some places within your body will feel dark while all the rest remains a golden color. The dark area within your body is a disease. Allow the light from the North Star to soak into this dark area until this place also becomes transparent. Then you will be charged with energy and your diseases will be healed.

It is unimportant that you are only using your imagination to practice this exercise — it works. "As you think, so will you be." You will find it helps to refresh, heal and strengthen your body. Whenever you have a disease, you may use this exercise to literally wash it away with the golden light. The best time to practice this meditation is in the evening when you are able to see the North Star clearly. However, it may be performed during the daytime by simply imagining that the star is there above you. However, always face the North when you are practicing the exercise. It will then be easy for your body to accept and receive the electromagnetic energy coming from the star. You may also find that the best position for your bed is to turn it so that it faces North. This way you will be in line with the natural lines of energy which surround the planet Earth.

CANDLELIGHT, SUNLIGHT AND MOONLIGHT CONTEMPLATIONS

If you are unable to locate the North Star, you may practice the exercise using a candle. Light the candle in a dark room and sit facing it. Close your eyes and imagine that you are pulling the golden light from the flame into your head. In a similar manner, you may use the sun or the moon as the source of the golden light which you wish to absorb into your body. Always imagine that you are pulling the light into your head and diffusing it throughout the body.

BRAIN CLEANSING BREATHING

The Brain Cleansing exercises utilize the Turtle, Deer and Crane breathing techniques to form the foundation upon which rests the Immortal Breathing. Without a firm foundation one cannot build a secure house which will be safe from winds of disease and negative mental attitudes. So before beginning any of the breathing techniques it is necessary to have practiced and to become proficient in combining the Deer, Crane and Turtle exercises.

We need to learn to relax not only the body, but the mind as well. Our minds are hosts to tremendous amounts of unnecessary worry which produces undue tension and stress and may lead to acute and chronic diseases. The Brain Cleansing Breathing is a basic healing technique which works to wash away stress from within our minds. Negative thoughts are large obstacles which prevent healing from occurring within our system. Taoism holds that an idea or thought *is* reality. Thus a negative thought cultivates a negative condition within our physical bodies. By practicing the Brain Cleansing exercises we gain a tool to empty the mind of all its useless thoughts, and bring it to a balanced state. If the mind is completely balanced so also will be the body. If you feel sick, this is an imbalance, but even if you feel well, this too is an imbalance. Taoism asks one to feel nothing to either extreme but just to *act naturally in the middle way*. We must awaken to our native condition and become empty to the point where there is neither positive or negative, neither hate or love — just an openness. Thus we become something great and nothing at all, at peace with ourselves.

> *Empty yourself of everything.*
> *Let the mind rest at peace.*
> *The ten thousand things rise and fall while the Self watches their*
> *return.*
> *They grow and flourish and then return to the source.*
> *Returning to the source is stillness, which is the way of nature.*
> *The way of nature is unchanging.*
> *Knowing constancy is insight.*
> *Not knowing constancy leads to disaster.*
> *Knowing constancy, the mind is open.*
> *With an open mind, you will be openhearted.*
> *Being openhearted, you will act royally.*
> *Being royal, you will attain the divine.*
> *Being divine, you will be at one with the Tao.*
> *Being at one with the Tao is eternal.*
> *And though the body dies, the Tao will never pass away.*

Tao Te Ching XVI

BRAIN CLEANSING ONE

The Brain Cleansing I breathing exercise begins in the Turtle sitting position. Sit with the back erect and with the hands resting lightly on the knees. Clasp the thumbs securely between the fingers. In this manner you hold onto the energy in your hands so that it recirculates back into the arms. Allow the eyes to remain closed throughout the exercise.

Now exhale all of the air from your lungs (without straining) as you assume the Turtle position with the head stretching upward and the shoulders down. Next, gently tilt the head backward into the second Turtle position and slowly begin to inhale the breath. Imagine in your mind's eye that as the breath enters into the internal chambers of your body it carries with it a boiling steam, fire or white smoke, and that it slowly begins to rise upward from the abdomen to the head. Imagine that the head completely fills with the visualization so the entire head becomes

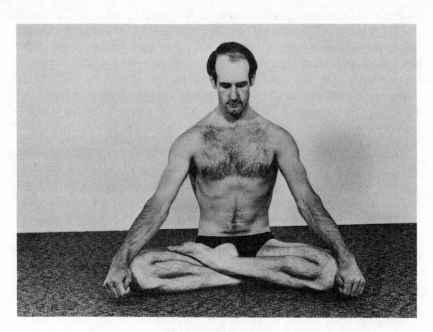

59. Brain Cleanse — One (1).

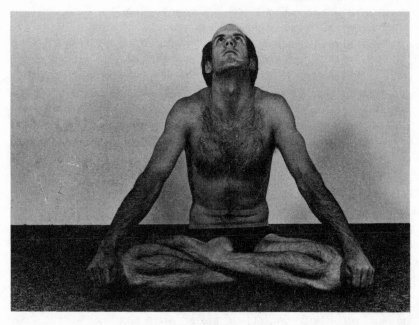

60. Brain Cleanse — One (2).

white. Become so that you cannot think, see or imagine anything but the white smoke, steam or fire which has filled the head.

When you have completed the inhalation (without straining), then straighten the head and begin to exhale in the first Turtle position. Exhale all the white smoke, steam or fire out of the body so that the head becomes empty. Imagine as the breath leaves the body, that it carries with it all your worries, tensions, unnecessary thoughts, bad traits such as dishonesty, anger, depression and ills of your mind and body. Imagine also as the smoke leaves your head, that it is replaced by a clear, clean and beautifully rich blue sky which leaves no room for worries or unclear thoughts. Then repeat the breathing sequence again as many times as you feel comfortable. However, try to maintain a minimum of seven inhalations and seven exhalations at each sitting.

At first it may be difficult to coordinate the breathing with the visualizations. But with determined and motivated practice, you will be able to clearly "see" the white smoke as it comes into and leaves your head. Also at first you may not be able to visualize the blue sky, but with patient practice you will be able to develop a very deep and beautiful blue color in your mind's eye. You will then have achieved a very great healing within yourself. The color blue will help to cleanse and purify the mind. If the mind is clear, then your problems will have been eighty percent eliminated.

It is important to remember to keep the anal muscles contracted while performing the Brain Cleansing exercise as this will lock the energy into the upper chambers of the body and will allow the energy and the smoke visualization to rise up the spine into the brain.

Negative thoughts are large obstacles which prevent healing from occurring within the body. The Brain Cleansing exercise helps to train the mind to become empty and to put it on an immortal level. Performing this breathing exercise will then be like catching a train as it passes by. The train is oneself and through this exercise the practitioner will be better able to understand his true nature. It will help one to come into harmony with the natural laws of the universe and prepare the mind for the next phase of Immortal Breathing. It will enable one to cast out of his mind limited concepts of wrong thinking and death and lead us to the edges of the Tao where there are no "isms" or dualistic thoughts, no desires, no diseases, but only complete peace.

BRAIN CLEANSING TWO

The Brain Cleansing II breathing exercise is performed while in a standing position (it may also be practiced from a prone position while lying on one's back) with the feet slightly apart but parallel to each other. The hands are relaxed but straight and are held at the sides of the body, and the head is in an upright position as in the first position of the Turtle exercise. Begin by exhaling the breath to completely empty the lungs. Now drop the head back and begin to inhale slowly. As you inhale, expand the chest and bring the arms up away from the sides of your body so that you bring the hands together up over your head with the palms together.

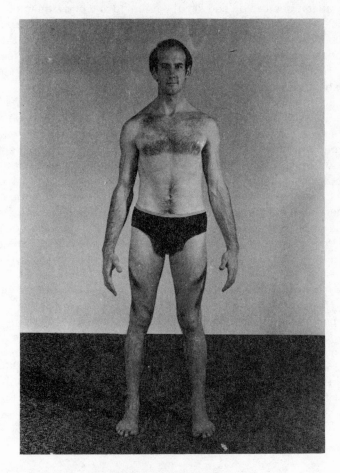

61. Brain Cleanse—Two (1).

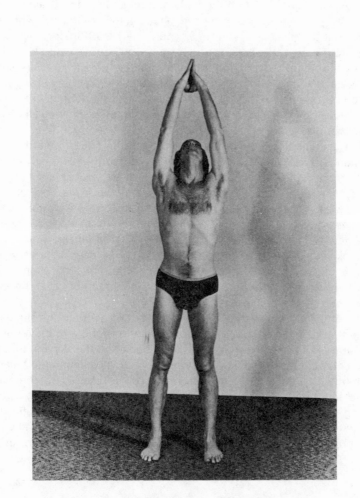

62. Brain Cleanse — Two (2).

(Do not strain during any of these movements. If it is impossible to touch the hands together comfortably, simply raise the hands as far as they will go and stop there.) As you bring the arms up over the head, feel as if you are bringing in the active (yang) energy of the universe into your lungs, body and mind. You may visualize in your mind's eye a white smoke, fire or a steam coming in to fill up the body and mind as in the Brain Cleansing I breathing exercise. After you have inhaled a full breath, and while still keeping the arms held over your head, hold the breath in, lock your anal muscles and relax in this pose for as long as you can without strain. Feel as if the white smoke is coming up to completely penetrate every space inside the mind so that you cannot see or think about anything else but the white cloud inside yourself. Feel the energy circulating around within your body and your mind, knowing that it is beginning to wash away all of your negative thoughts.

Next, as you slowly begin to exhale, bring the head forward, separate the hands; keeping the arms straight, move them back down to your sides. As your hands move in the downward arc, try to visualize the passive (yin) energy from the earth coming into the arms through your fingers. This exercise is symbolic of embracing the entire universe so that one achieves a feeling of oneness from uniting the earthly passive energy with the active, heavenly energy. As you continue to exhale, imagine the white smoke coming out of the body and being replaced by a very rich, blue sky inside your head; when you have finished exhaling, then repeat the breathing and arm movement sequence a minimum of seven times or until you feel like stopping.

It is refreshing to practice this exercise out of doors in the sunshine, gathering the fresh air into the body. As you perform the arm movements, feel as if you are reaching out to touch the clouds and the sky and that the rich blue color comes in to fill up your mind. As well as helping to balance one's energy, this exercise provides a marvelous stretch to the back, shoulders and arms and relieves tension and fatigue from the body as well as helping to keep the mind alert and fresh. It is therefore beneficial to practice the Brain Cleansing II exercise at any time during the day when you feel tired, such as in the morning upon arising, at the office or in the evening after work.

5 Immortal Breathing: Small Heavenly Cycle

The seven glands of the human body (corresponding to the subtle energy centers, or *chakras*), are responsible for controlling all of the bodily functions. They include the sexual glands, adrenals, pancreas, thymus, thyroid, pituitary and pineal gland. These seven glands mutually balance and are interconnected with one another. They energize, recharge and help circulate energy in the body and may be likened to electrical transformers or generators or storehouses of energy within the human body. When the seven houses are full of life (energy) and their functioning is perfert, then the entire body will be in a perfect or spiritual order.

Before undertaking the Immortal Breathing, it is necessary that one must have already achieved sufficient expertise in the system of Internal Exercises so that the body is in a balanced state of health without any serious or chronic ailments. It is impossible to practice the final stages of the breathing exercises if there are any blockages in the meridian pathways. The Meridian Meditation and the other Internal Exercises therefore are necessary prerequisites for opening up the meridians and preparing the body for receiving the Immortal Breath.

The human body is an electrical system. It is capable of carrying a load of electricity through it only as strong as the resistance of the nerves and glands are to that electrical current. The stronger the body is physically, the greater the current load of electricity it will be able to handle. Immortal breathing brings into the body very powerful levels of energy and if the body is not sufficiently strong to handle it, the nerves and glands may "burn out" from an overload of energy. It has been said that many people who suffer from extreme mental conditions are that way only because they are unable to handle the energy levels flowing within their bodies. Unfortunately, if one experiences excessively high levels of energy over too long a period of time, irreversible damage may be done to the body. *Do not, therefore, undertake Immortal Breathing lightly.* However, if you have followed the steps of the Internal Exercises conscientiously and have practiced the Crane, Turtle and Deer exercises so that you are proficient in them, and have mastered the Meridian Meditation so that you are clearly able to feel the circulation of energy throughout your body and have no blockages within your meridian channels, and if your desires and motives are clear and pure, then you are ready to begin the Immortal Breathing.

This is the final stage of the Taoist system of Internal Exercises. Mastery of Immortal Breathing may require from one year to a lifetime of diligent practice. Through its practice, the energy of the body is raised until all of the seven houses are operating at their full capacity. At this point the spiritual eye of the practitioner is fully awakened and he or she is raised to the level of the *Hsien* or wise and immortal person, one who knows the secrets of the universe by continuously being in touch with the natural laws which guide him or her in daily life. At this level, one has awakened to the true Self and understands the order of the Tao by being one with it. He or she has achieved total union within himself or herself and has thus come to know his or her true place in the universal order of life. Is this not the true desire which lies in the hearts of all men?

> My words are easy to understand and easy to perform.
> Yet no man under heaven knows them or practices them.
> My words have ancient beginnings.
> My actions are disciplined.
> Because men do not understand, they have no knowledge of me.
> Those that know me are few.
> Those that abuse me are honored.
> Therefore the sage wears rough clothing and holds the jewel in
>   his heart.

Tao Te Ching LXX

SMALL HEAVENLY CYCLE

Assume a sitting position with your spine and head held erect. Grasp the thumbs inside the fingers and lay the hands lightly on the legs. Begin to inhale slowly (without forcing the breath at any time). As you inhale, allow the breath to come in through the nose and descend through the Jen-Mo meridian into the abdominal cavity (stove) where the breath will be heated (transmuted) and energized. When you have fully inhaled the breath, lock your anal and sphincter muscles and pull the chin down into the chest in a chin lock. These two movements prevent the energy from escaping the abdominal chamber and help to further energize the energy as it activates the sexual glands. Also, when you hold your breath, the blood vessels tend to constrict, thus raising the blood pressure. The chin lock helps to reverse this process and restore an equilibrium to the body.

With the breath held, and the anal and chin locks in place, begin to visualize and feel the energy in the stove cauldron (abdomen) beginning to rise upward along the back of the spinal column or Tu-Mo meridian. As it travels upward, it moves through the seven houses (glands) in succession, entering first into the sexual glands where it makes a spiraling circular movement, and then passes upward and through the remaining six houses in similar wheel-like movements (see Figure A). The wheel rotations at each house serve to energize the house in which it occurs, as well as transform the energy into a higher order to be received by the next

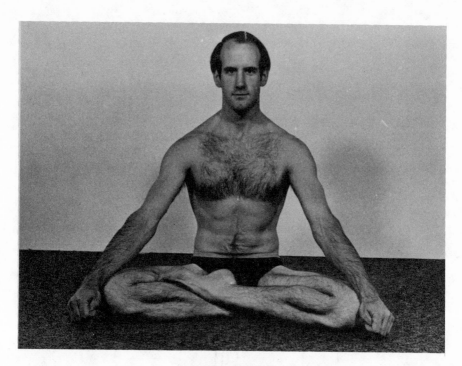

63. Sitting Pose (1).

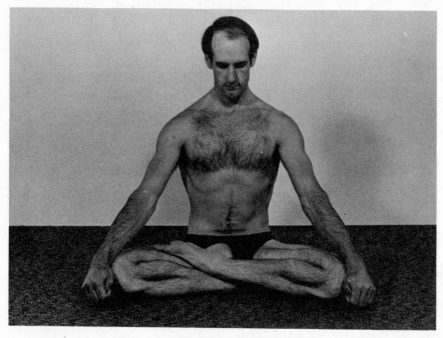

64. Sitting Pose (2).

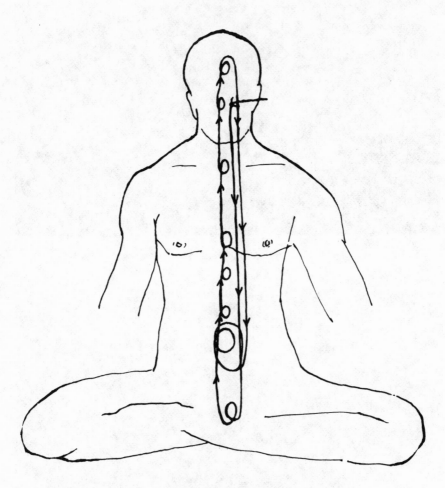

Fig. 24.   The Small Heavenly Cycle.

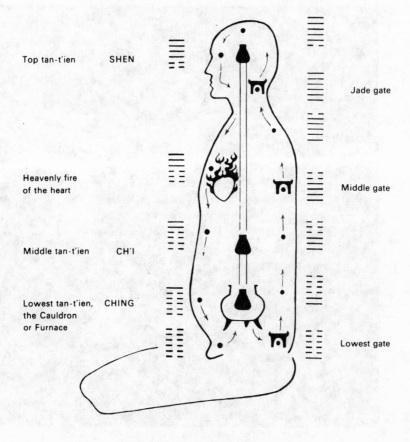

Top tan-t'ien   SHEN

Jade gate

Heavenly fire
of the heart

Middle gate

Middle tan-t'ien   CH'I

Lowest tan-t'ien,   CHING
the Cauldron
or Furnace

Lowest gate

Fig. 25.   Fire of Eternal Life

123

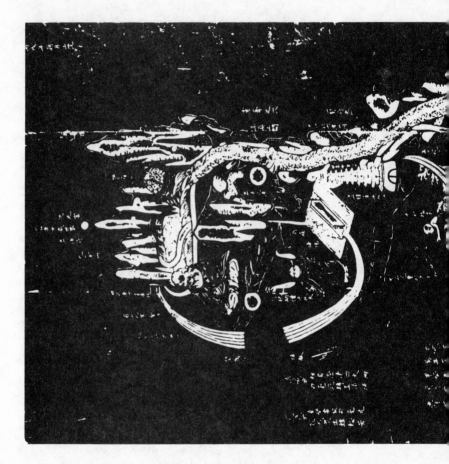

124

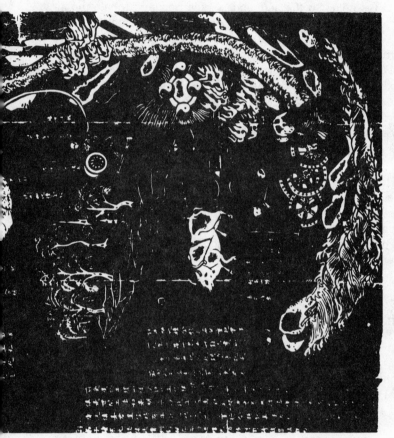

Diagram of the Subtle body, mapping the Inner Alchemy. Rubbing dated 1886, Ch'ing dynasty.

house. In this fashion each of the glands serves as transformer and generator for the energy of the body.

When the energy has reached up into the pineal gland, allow it to circulate there for a moment, and then release the anal and chin locks and slowly exhale the breath. Then begin the Small Heavenly Cycle again.

At first, you will want to hold the breath only for seven seconds, one second for each gland. As you become proficient in the breathing, hold the breath for longer periods of time. As the breath is held for longer periods, begin to make two or more loops around the houses for each period during which the breath is held. So the sequence would become: Inhale the air into the abdomen through the Jen-Mo meridian; hold the breath and lock the chin and anal muscles; pass the energy up and through the Tu-Mo meridian into the sexual glands, adrenals, pancreas, thymus, thyroid, pituitary and pineal glands then back down the Jen-Mo, and so on until there is the need to exhale the breath. With practice the breath can be held for several minutes to several hours without feeling the need to breathe. When the seven houses have been sufficiently energized, the need to breathe disappears and one functions in a breathless state of immortality.

This type of breathing is often called the "self-winding wheel of the law." When first practicing this type of breathing, one must use one's will power to initiate the cycle. However, there comes a time when the breathing becomes automatic and will continue on an involuntary basis. Thus, once the process has been initiated, it becomes something which in a manner of speaking, becomes self-winding, irreversible and beyond your control. In such a way the final stage of enlightenment comes not from something you are doing, but comes all of its own to you.

LARGE HEAVENLY CYCLE

The Large Heavenly Cycle, like the Small Heavenly Cycle, utilizes the breath and the seven basic houses (glands) of the body. The difference between the two techniques is that the Large Heavenly Cycle allows the energy to travel down the meridians of the legs and arms in addition to the central axial chamber of the body.

Begin in a seated position with the spine and head held erect. Inhale the breath and allow it to pass through the Jen-Mo meridian in the front of the body to the abdominal cauldron (stove) where it will be fired up and energized. After a full inhalation, perform the chin and anal lock, hold the breath, and allow the energy to circulate through the seven houses (as described in the Small Heavenly Cycle). When the energy has reached the pineal glands, allow it to descend again down the Jen-Mo meridian into the legs through the stomach, bladder and gallbladder meridians which lie along the outside of the legs. When the energy has reached the toes, bring it back up your legs through the spleen-pancreas, kidney and liver meridians which lie along the inside of the legs. Circulate the energy back up the spine along the Tu-Mo meridian and then allow it to descend down the arms through the lung, heart and heart constrictor meridians which lie along the inside of each arm. When the energy has reached the finger tips, allow the energy to pass back up the arms through the large intestine, small intestine and triple heater meridians and bring it back into the Jen-Mo meridian and down to the abdominal cauldron. This completes one Large Heavenly Cycle. You may now exhale the breath or continue to perform the breathing cycle until you feel the need to exhale the breath.

Begin the exercise by holding the breath for seven seconds while leading the energy around your body. With increased proficiency, increase the time to five minutes or more and perform as many rotations of the large cycle as possible, always ending the breath with the energy in the abdominal cauldron. You may eventually reach the point where there is no need felt to inhale or exhale the breath. It is at this level that the cells of the body have been transmuted through an alchemical process to where they are able to exist only on the energy which circulates throughout the universe rather than on the grosser need for oxygen which is presently felt. It is at this point that the "normal" laws of time and space no longer bind the individual to this body or earth and one has entered into the eternal nature of the universe, from which all knowledge, understanding and peace emanate. In this way, the law of the Tao is fulfilled.

6 *Taoist Healing Prescriptions*

The Internal Energizing Exercises may be divided into four distinct categories: 1) general and regular health maintenance exercises; 2) specific healing exercises for individual organs or parts of the body; 3) breathing exercises; and 4) contemplative techniques. In addition, there are healing prescriptions which combine several of the Internal Exercise techniques and are used when treating a specific disease or ailment.

The general health maintenance exercises are to be practiced on a daily basis for a minimum of three months. Then one should continue to practice the Deer, Crane and Turtle daily, and use the other exercises on a schedule of alternate days or weeks so as to build the body to its maximum level of health. It will take between three months and one year to feel the health-enhancing benefits which these exercises will bring to the practitioner. After about three months one should be able to feel the flow of energy in the body as one practices these exercises. When one can perceive this subtle flow of energy or life force (Chi or Qi) within the body, then it will be time to begin practicing the Meridian Meditation techniques. To properly learn the contemplative exercises takes between one and ten years. Develop patience in your practice and you will be rewarded. Practicing the Taoist Internal Exercises is like venturing into a dark cave and discovering a treasure which has been lying there for years waiting its discovery. Upon returning to the sunlight, that treasure will sparkle magnificently. The treasure is your health and the Taoists feel that perfect health is our birthright.

You may find from time to time that you will go through periods when you are unable to perform your exercises (because of location, family or political crises, etc.). If you have become genuinely interested and are able to see the benefits you will have accrued from doing the Internal Exercises up to that point, have faith that you will return and begin again where you left off. The Internal Exercise system is to be practiced throughout one's lifetime. Therefore, minor periods when one does not practice them will be insignificant if one follows them for the bulk of one's lifetime.

The constitutions of some people upon beginning the Internal Exercises may be every weak, or there may be chronic problems which have been developing over the years. Even if one practices the exercises, whether because of poor diet or an excess of stress in one's daily life or through injury, one may acquire diseases or problems of health such as heart disease, obesity, or lower back pain. Included in the system of Internal Exercises, therefore, are techniques designed to deal with specific problems of the body. These are prescribed on an individual level, and are to be practiced until the disease, pain, or problem disappears entirely. They are to be practiced in conjunction with the other general health maintenance exercises.

Included in this chapter are also healing prescription or combinations of several Internal Exercises which, when practiced together, aid the natural healing processes in certain states of discomfort or disease such as migraine headache, high blood pressure or hemorrhoids.

General Health Maintenance Schedule

Upon waking in the morning:

    Toe wiggling and body stretch

    Internal organ relaxation

    Head rubbing

    Healing and strengthening the eyes

    The nose, lungs and sinuses

    Beating the Heavenly Drum

    Mouth exercises

    Rubbing the face

    Stimulating the kidneys

    Liver exercise

    Bringing fire into the stove

    Rubbing the arms and legs

    Deer

    Crane

    Turtle

Regular Health Maintenance

To be done daily throughout one's life:

    Deer

    Crane

    Turtle

Meditation

Upon feeling the subtle energy flow in the body one may begin practicing the meditation:

    Meridian Meditation

Only after mastering the Meridian Meditation should one begin to practice the Immortal Breathing techniques.

Specific Healing Exercises

These may be practiced in conjunction with the general health maintenance exercises or just for curing specific ailments:

Weight reducing exercises

Lower back strengthening exercise

Stomach disease curing exercise

Heart exercise

Heart energizing exercise

Abdominal strengthening exercise

Lung energizing exercise

Leg and sexual gland stimulating exercise

Pain relief exercise

Hand and arm pressing exercise

Arm exercises

Sun worship exercise

Eye exercises

Internal organ relaxation

Complete relaxation exercises and bone breathing

Breathing Exercises Include:

Crane exercise

Brain Cleanse One

Brain Cleanse Two

Immortal Breathing
Small Heavenly Cycle
Large Heavenly Cycle

HEALING PRESCRIPTIONS

Arthritis, Rheumatism, Bursitis:

Turtle
Crane
Deer
Arm and leg stimulating exercises
Hand pressing (for bursitis or arthritis in arms or hands)

Tennis Elbow:

Turtle
Pain relief exercise
Hand pressing
Arm stimulating exercises (rub until you feel the arm becoming hot around the elbow — use visualization to imagine a fire coming into the elbow to produce this heat)

Asthma:

> Crane, Turtle, Deer — all practiced together
> Lung exercise
> Liver exercise (soothes and strengthens the nerves)

Back Pain:

> Lower back strengthening exercise
> Kidney exercise

Beauty and Fitness (rejuvenation):

> Deer, Crane, Turtle
> Eye exercises (for wrinkles)
> Teeth and gum exercises
> Drinking the heavenly water
> Beating the heavenly drum
> Teeth clicking
> Weight reducing exercises
> Head rubbing

Blood Pressure — High:

> Crane, Turtle
> Brain Cleanse One
> Toe wiggling
> (Avoid Deer exercise until pressure falls to normal)

Blood Pressure — Low:

> Deer, Turtle
> Brain Cleanse One
> Toe wiggling
> (Avoid Crane until pressure comes up)

Bronchitis (throat pains):

> Lung exercises
> Arm rubbing (especially downward along lung meridian)
> Clockwise rubbing of abdomen (disperses blockage out of body)

Cancer (prevention):

> Crane, Turtle, Deer
> Arm stimulating exercises
> Kneading shoulder muscles (releases tension and stress and opens
> meridians which may be blocked)

> *Bone cancer:*
>
>> Kidney exercise
>> Lower back exercise
>> Pancreas and liver exercise

Cellulite:

> Leg stimulating exercises (rub downward on outside only)
> Leg and sex gland exercise

Common Cold (sneezing, coughing, sinus headache):

Internal organ relaxation (brings blood into head and lungs to fight head cold)

Nose pressing exercises (for sinus)

Press points behind head (for headache and tension)

For coughing press on either side of the throat on the stomach meridian. This may cause you to cough at first, but will eventually stop the coughing.

Arm rubbing (downward along lung meridian for temporary relief of cold symptoms and lung congestion)

Constipation:

Crane breathing

Abdominal rubbing (clockwise for dispersion)

Press on large intestine with firm and hard pressure and rotate in a clockwise direction

Diabetes:

Liver and pancreas rubbing exercise

Leg stimulating exercise (especially upward on inside of leg to bring energy into the body)

Deer exercise

(For relief of symptoms of thirst caused by diabetes, drink the heavenly water.)

Diarrhea:

Deer exercise

Leg stimulating exercise on inside of leg, rubbing in an upward motion only

Abdominal rubbing in *counterclockwise* motion

Dizziness (vertigo, nerve imbalance):

Bone breathing

Ear exercise

Brain Cleanse Two

Turtle, Crane

Emphysema:

See Asthma

Eye Problems (glaucoma, cataract, near- and far-sightedness, etc.):

Eye exercises

Female Problems:

Deer with breast rubbing

Kidney exercise

Leg stimulating exercise on inside of legs only

Abdominal rubbing (both directions)

Headache:

> Bone Breathing
> Eye exercises
> Nose exercises
> Standing Crane
> Brain Cleanse Two
> Rub points behind the head (especially painful ones)

Hearing Problems:

> Ear exercises

Heart Problems:

> Heart exercise

Hepatitis (liver problems):

> Liver exercise

Hemorrhoids:

> Deer exercise (squeezing anal muscles)
> Sunworship exercise

Impotence (premature ejaculation):

> Deer
> Brain Cleanse One
> Sex gland stimulation

Insomnia:

> Toe wiggling
> Crane breathing
> Bone breathing
> Abdominal rubbing (both directions)

Kidney Problems:

> Kidney exercise
> Deer
> Leg stimulating (upward on inside only)

Menstrual Problems:

> See Female Problems

Nerve Problems (numbness and paralysis). See also Liver Problems:

> Crane, Deer and Turtle exercises
> Liver exercise
> Rub local area until warm using visualization to bring in fresh blood
> and energy.

Obesity:

> Weight reducing exercise
> Abdominal rubbing exercise

Overacidity:

    Crane

    Liver exercise (calms and balances stomach)

Pneumonia:

    Crane breathing (to help rest lungs, very slowly)

    Rub downward along lung meridian (for temporary relief)

Prostate Problems:

    Deer exercise

Refreshing Yourself:

    Deer, Crane and Turtle

    Bone breathing

    Internal organ relaxation

    Eye exercises

Sciatica:

    Leg stimulating exercise

    Lower back exercise

    Leg and sex gland stimulation

Stomach Problems (ulcers, pain, vomiting). See also Diarrhea:

    Crane

    Stomach exercises

Stomach Problems (nausea from hypoglycemia):

    Liver exercise

    Rub across pancreas

Tennis Elbow:

    See Arthritis

Teeth and Gums:

    Teeth clicking

    Gum exercises

Tonsilitis:

    Turtle

    Throat rubbing

Tuberculosis:

    Crane

    Coughing complications:

        Rub down inside of arms

        Throat rubbing

    Sweating complications:

        Toe wiggling (calming)

    Diarrhea complications:

        Abdominal rubbing counterclockwise

        Crane, Deer exercises

Ulcer:

See Stomach Problems and Nerve Problems

Vomiting:

Crane exercise
Stomach exercises

7 *In Summary*

When thinking about integrating the system of Internal Exercises into our daily lives, it is important to keep in mind the ancient Taoist proverb which states simply: "If you do external exercises, you *must* do internal exercises." External exercises expend energy without replacing it and therefore we feel a need to rest after strenuous physical activity. On the other hand, Internal Exercises work to conserve and build up our energy. The proverb continues: "If you do internal exercises, you may forget to practice external exercises" — because one benefits completely through the practice of internal exercises.

This is not to imply that one should not practice external exercises such as tennis, running or golf. The Taoists were only recognizing the fact that, by themselves, external exercises are incomplete and need to be balanced by the addition of these simple techniques for rebalancing and supplanting the loss of energy incurred through external exercises.

The Internal Exercises energize, train and strengthen the internal organs and tissues so they become strong and healthy. When the internal body and mind is strong, we will lack the opportunity to become diseased. The beauty of the Internal Exercises is that they are very easy to practice. No matter where you are or what time it is, it is possible to practice these simple techniques. When you are on the toilet, practice the eye exercises; when you are driving along in your car, do the Deer exercise by squeezing the sphincter muscles. Nothing could be simpler or easier to practice; no special equipment is needed and no one else need know what you are doing!

In addition, Internal Exercises encourage the circulatory system without speeding up the heart rate. All the exercises are done slowly, without effort. The heart is like an engine that has a definite life expectancy. From around the second week after our conception to the moment we die, our heart continues to beat. Therefore we can say that the number of times our heart beats during our lifetime indicates the length of our life. We do not want the heart to wear out prematurely. One of the fundamental principles behind the Internal Exercises is that the heart rate does not increase during the practice of the exercises, and yet, through their practice, the heart rate slows down. We are therefore able to increase our life expectancy as the ancient Taoists wished.

Oftentimes, people who practice external exercises become involved in a subtle, yet destructive cycle. External exercises work to train the muscular system. Vigorous exercise often stimulates the appetite and the person in training ends up eating more than he or she would otherwise. All goes well until the person stops exercising, and then all the muscles which have been built up turn to fatty tissues. *This does not occur through the practice of the Internal Exercises.* They work to control the size and tightness of the muscles and other tissues without encouraging the appetite. As a matter of fact, many report that the Turtle exercise actually decreases their appetite.

The ancient Taoists recognized that the Internal Exercises follow natural laws in working to fulfill their final purpose. Will power is not necessary to practice these exercises, for one is not interested in making impossible things occur, only in doing what is possible. By practicing the Internal Exercises, one forgets oneself and the ego becomes smaller, while the spirit or god within becomes larger.

There are four kingdoms within this world. The first, or vegetable kingdom, has no purpose other than to exist and grow; plants have no mind of their own. The second, or animal kingdom, has mind and soul, but lacks a spirit and therefore has no purpose other than to propagate itself. The third realm, the kingdom of man, has mind, soul and spirit. If we ask why man has religion, we realize that man is not content with his situation as it is. Animals do not seem to care about their situation, but man does. He has a higher purpose than merely to exist. This is exemplified in man's pursuit of his material life — he always wants something more than he has. We also have a desire to improve ourselves. Why? Because we have a spiritual need to improve ourselves into the kingdom of God. To be religious means to find a way to get into the divine kingdom of God, the fourth realm of this universe — to become immortal. The ancient Taoists recognized this primal urge of mankind and through their knowledge of the natural laws perfected this system of Internal Exercises as a means whereby — with daily practice — man could realize his birthright, his divine self. The system of Internal Exercise is meant to provide each of us with the opportunity to unify our bodies with our minds and our spiritual selves. Only then can we realize the Tao, our true immortality, and enter into the kingdom of God.